The Art of Healing Crystals

The Illustrated Guide to Discovering the Benefits of the Top 40 Crystals. Learn how to rebalance the Chakras and heal Mind, Soul, and Body.

Ambra Keller

Copyright © 2023 – Ambra Keller

All rights reserved.

This paper is geared toward providing accurate and reliable information regarding the subject matter and issue covered. The publication is sold with the idea that the publisher is not required to provide accounting, officially licensed, or otherwise qualified services if advice is needed, legal or professional, a licensed individual should be appointed. It is in no way legal to reproduce, duplicate or transmit any part of this document in electronic or printed form. Recording of this publication is strictly prohibited, and storage of this document is not permitted except with the written permission of the publisher. All rights reserved. The information provided herein is declared to be true and consistent in that any liability, in terms of carelessness or otherwise, from any use or misuse of any policy, process, or direction contained within is the solitary and absolute responsibility of the recipient reader. In no event shall any legal liability or fault be taken against the publisher for any redress, damage, or monetary loss due to the information contained herein, directly or indirectly. The information contained herein is provided for informational purposes only and is universal. The presentation of the information is without a contract or any type of warranty. Trademarks used within this book are for clarification purposes only and are the property of the owners themselves, not affiliated with this document.

Summary:

Introduction..7
What is Crystal Healing...9
    The stones and the different colors................................10
    Crystal structure..12
Zodiac signs and Chakras..15
    Zodiac signs..13
    Chakras and Colors..19
Purifying, Charging and Using crystals..............................23
    Purifying the stones...23
    Recharge crystals and energize them..............................25
    How to use crystals...27
Guide to crystals..29
    Aquamarine..32
    Agata...34
    Amazonite...36
    Amber...38
    Amethyst..40
    Green aventurine..42
    Carnelian..44
    Diamond...46
    Diaspro...48
    Hematite..50
    Fluorite...52
    Fuchsite...54
    Jade...56

Garnet..58
Howlite...60
Labradorite..62
Lapislazuli..64
Larimar...66
Magnetite..68
Malachite...70
Moldavite...72
Tiger's eye..74
Onix..76
Fire opal...78
Obsidian snowflake..80
Moonstone..82
Citrine quartz..84
Smoked quartz...86
Rose quartz..88
Rhodochrosite..90
Rubin..92
Selenite..94
Emerald..96
Sodalite..98
Tanzanite...100
Topaz..102
Green tourmaline..104
Turquoise...106
Sapphire...108
Zircon..110
Conclusion..113

Introduction

This guide introduces you to the fascinating world of crystals and gemstones. Crystal therapy is not a magical solution, but it can help you restore your energy balance and deal with your problems in a more peaceful way. Ultimately, this guide gives you an overview of the world of crystals and gemstones and can help you discover new tools for your well-being. However, it is important to always keep in mind that crystal therapy is not a substitute for traditional medical treatment and that it is always advisable to consult your physician before using any type of alternative therapy.

What is crystal healing

Crystal healing falls under holistic disciplines and is an ancient alternative medicine technique that uses stones and crystals to promote self-knowledge and well-being. Everything in the universe is made of atoms, which have a nucleus composed of protons and neutrons and are surrounded by one or more vibrating electrons. These vibrations are the electromagnetic force that forms everything we see. We human beings are also made of atoms, as are crystals. When a vibrating system is stimulated with similar frequencies, the phenomenon of resonance occurs. In essence, our bodies and everything around us are made of vibrating matter that can affect each other through vibrational resonance.

Each crystal emanates an energy field that is attuned to the wearer's energy field, producing different effects. Crystal therapy is based on this principle, as the vibrations of crystals have the power to amplify, calm or give new energy, stimulating self-healing processes and developing awareness. The energies of living beings are subtle and interact with the cosmos and the environment around us through gateways called chakras.

The chakras are the energy centers of our bodies, and sometimes they work disharmoniously, generating problems; mastering the art of crystal therapy can rebalance the energy.

The stones and the different colors

- **Black stones**: black crystals have the property of absorbing excess energy, promoting healing, and working on the first chakra. Not recommended when you are already out of energy, these crystals can be used when you feel the need to connect to your roots or to one's ancestors.

- **Red stones**: bring warmth to life, stimulate feelings and emotions, and have great energy. Useful for strengthening character, self-esteem, creativity, and the will to strive to achieve goals. These crystals are associated with the first chakra and are useful for giving concreteness and rationality.

- **White stones**: symbolize purity, hope, and trust and are related to the seventh chakra.

- **Purple stones**: stimulate memory and work on the sixth chakra, located between the eyebrows. Purple represents magic, mystery, and spirituality and symbolizes creativity and intellect.

- **Yellow stones**: represent light and are related to the third chakra, stimulating creativity and positivity. The yellow is associated with the strength to have new experiences.

- **Orange stones**: symbolize vitality, energy, and inner harmony. Orange is useful against depression and psychological illnesses, helping to overcome trauma.

- **Pink stones**: represent tender love, understanding, and insight and are related to the fourth chakra.

- **Gray stones**: –symbolize detachment, prudence, and wisdom and are the fusion of the primary colors black and white.

- **Green stones**: stimulate pure feelings and positive emotions, releasing pent-up anger. They are related to the fourth chakra and represent good fortune, balance, and harmony.

- **Blue stones**: stimulate honesty and induce following the sixth sense, working on the fifth throat chakra. Blue is used to ward off anxiety and stabilize the heartbeat.

Crystal structure

There are seven types of crystal structures, each with its own particular characteristics, and we can find affinities with them according to our personality:

- <u>Cubic system</u>: their internal structure is based on the square shape. The meaning of these stones reflects this order and indicates a love of control, rules, and, indeed, order.

- <u>Hexagonal system</u>: their internal structure has six faces. Good for people characterized by analytical thinking and who are not deterred by difficulties.

- <u>Trigonal system</u>: their internal structure has three faces. Perfect for those who are quiet of spirit and always try to avoid conflicts and disputes with others.

- <u>Tetragonal system</u>: these crystals indicate a love of novelty and are recommended for those who hate monotony and routine and are always seeking new experiences.

- <u>Rhombic system</u>: –from the name, the internal structure of these stones is rhombic, as occurs in peridot and topaz. These gemstones are aligned with the thinking of some who have a linear view of life in which obstacles should be as few as possible.

- <u>Monoclinic system</u>: parallelogram internal structure and are suitable for those who do not like to make long-term plans but prefer to seize the moment.

- <u>Triclinic system</u>: trapezoidal internal structure and are perfect for those who are spontaneous every day.

- <u>Amorphous system</u>: all exceptions to the rule, i.e., all stones that do not have a defined crystal structure, belong to this category; they are a perfect match for those who are happy to deal with new things and for those who lead versatile lifestyles.

Zodiac signs and Chakras

Zodiac signs:

Aries
The zodiac sign of Aries begins with the arrival of spring (March 21-April 20) and is characterized by the element of fire and the presence of the planet Mars. These astrological influences give those born under this sign a passionate, sincere, optimistic, and stubborn personality. The colors associated with this sign are deep red, orange, and gold.

Taurus
The zodiac sign Taurus, which runs from April 21 to May 20, is characterized by the earth element and the planet Venus. People born under this sign are known for their stubborn and determined nature and are inclined to love material possessions and to go on until the end, struggling persistently to achieve what they desire. The colors associated with this sign are green and dark brown.

Gemini

The sign of Gemini (May 21-June 21) is characterized by the element air and the planet Mercury, which gives people born under this sign a lively intelligence and great curiosity. They are communicative, sociable, and adaptable but can sometimes be shallow and unstable. The colors associated with this sign are yellow and blue.

Cancer

People born under the sign of Cancer (June 22-July 22), ruled by the Moon and the water element, are very protective of the things they consider important, especially when it comes to their personal space and intimacy. Their attitude can sometimes lead them to isolate themselves. The colors associated with this sign are silver, white, and pearl gray.

Leo

Ruled by the sun and the element of fire, the sign of Leo (July 23-Aug. 22) is naturally strong, outgoing, and vital. Always the center of attention, those born under this sign often tend to dominate. The colors associated with this sign are gold, orange, and red.

Virgo

Those born under the sign of Virgo (Aug. 23-Sept. 22) are characterized by the earth element and the planet Mercury; they are precise, detail-oriented, and workaholics.

However, their perfectionism can lead them to be far too demanding of themselves and others. The colors associated with this sign are beige, gray, and brown.

Libra

Those born under the sign of Libra (Sept. 23-Oct. 23), a sign ruled by the planet Venus and the element air, are known for their aversion to conflict, their objectivity, and their fairness. They are often indecisive but can always find the right words at the right times. The colors associated with this sign are pink, blue, and green.

Scorpio

Those born under the sign of Scorpio (Oct. 24-Nov. 21) are characterized by the water element and the planets Mars and Pluto, are deep and mysterious, and often tend toward introspection. When they feel attacked, they may overreact. They are very intelligent and cannot stand superficial people or frivolous relationships, always looking for the hidden meaning of any friendship or romance. The colors associated with this sign are black, red, and burgundy.

Sagittarius

Those born under the sign of Sagittarius (Nov. 22-Dec. 21), ruled by the planet Jupiter and the element of fire, do not know how to sit still: whether it is sports, training the mind, or solving a problem right away, these people love adventure and are often impulsive in their choices. The colors associated with this sign are purple, blue, and burgundy.

Capricorn

People born under the sign of Capricorn (Dec. 22-Jan. 19) are characterized by the earth element and the planet Saturn; they are shy by nature, and it is not easy for them to bond with others. However, when they manage to do so, they become extremely affectionate and helpful. They are known for their seriousness and ambition. The colors associated with this sign are brown, black, and gray.

Aquarius

People born under the sign of Aquarius (Jan. 20-Feb. 19) are characterized by the air element and the planets Uranus and Saturn; they are selfless and seek to improve the lives of others. They love to make decisions independently and are stimulated by novelty. They do not show excessive attachment but sacrifice themselves for their loved ones. They love solitude and routine. The colors associated with this sign are blue and turquoise.

Pisces

People born under the sign of Pisces (Feb. 20-March 20), ruled by the planet Neptune and the water element, are good-hearted, sensitive, and introverted. They are quiet and open but tend to be affected by negative experiences; however, they always manage to be a source of inspiration for others and often find expression through art. The colors associated with this sign are purple, pink, and green.

Chakras and colors

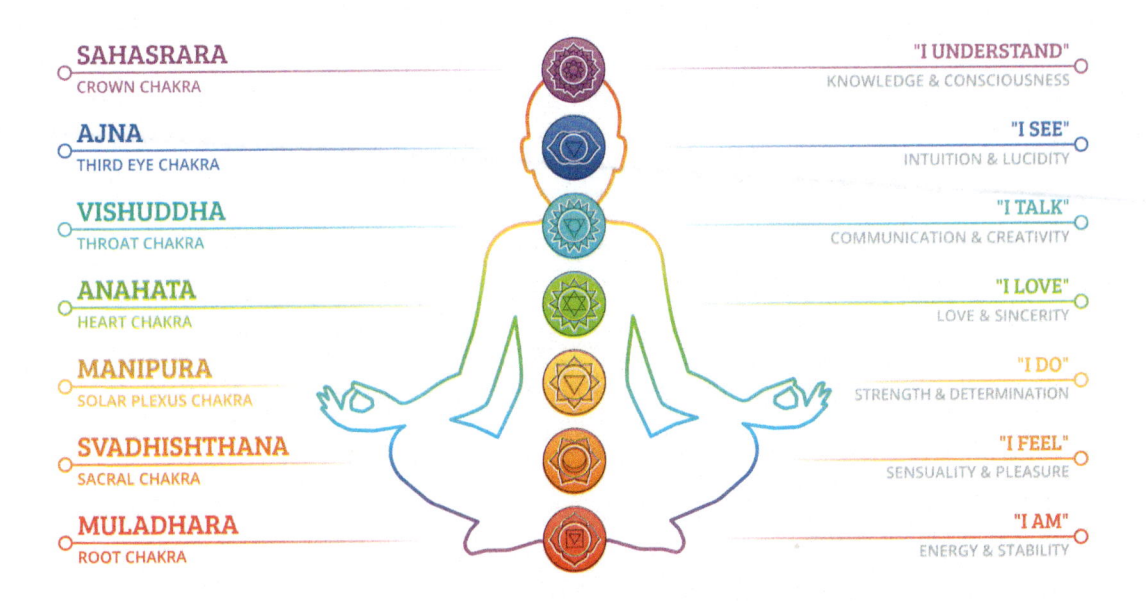

SAHASRARA — CROWN CHAKRA		"I UNDERSTAND" — KNOWLEDGE & CONSCIOUSNESS
AJNA — THIRD EYE CHAKRA		"I SEE" — INTUITION & LUCIDITY
VISHUDDHA — THROAT CHAKRA		"I TALK" — COMMUNICATION & CREATIVITY
ANAHATA — HEART CHAKRA		"I LOVE" — LOVE & SINCERITY
MANIPURA — SOLAR PLEXUS CHAKRA		"I DO" — STRENGTH & DETERMINATION
SVADHISHTHANA — SACRAL CHAKRA		"I FEEL" — SENSUALITY & PLEASURE
MULADHARA — ROOT CHAKRA		"I AM" — ENERGY & STABILITY

The chakras are energy centers distributed along the spine and reaching all the way up to the top of the head, and they have the function of distributing energy to both our physique and our mind.

In the lowest part of the spine resides kundalini, the tangled energy in the form of a snake that must awaken and rise up, forming a kind of spiral passing through all seven chakras.

It is essential to balance these energy centers in order to live in harmony with ourselves and get in touch with consciousness.

Starting from the base of the spine, we will have:

The first chakra
Muladhara or root chakra, is the foundation of the body's energy system and is represented by the color red and the element earth. Located in the perineum, it controls the lymphatic system, the sense of smell, the lower extremities, and the bone system. On a mental level, this chakra governs our stability and sense of security, but it can be blocked by fear. Its malfunction can lead to guilt, shyness, fear, distraction, distrust, and dependence on material goods.

The second chakra
Svadhisthana or sacral chakra, is represented by the color orange and the element water. Located in the center of the abdomen, about two fingers below the navel, it is connected to the sexual organs and governs freedom of expression, creativity, and pleasure. Guilt can block this energy center, leading to fear of enjoyment, disdain for sex, and sexual repression.

The third chakra
Manipura or solar plexus chakra, is represented by the color yellow and the element fire. Located just below the diaphragm in the solar plexus, it involves the liver, stomach, muscular system, and skin, but also personal power, confidence, and willpower. It is blocked by shame, and its malfunction can cause symptoms such as weight on the stomach, acidity, ulcers, self-centeredness, a sense of inferiority, guilt, and personal dissatisfaction.

The fourth chakra
Anahata or heart chakra, is represented by the color green and is associated with the element air. It is located at chest height, in the center, and controls the circulatory system, lungs, heart, and the entire chest area. It governs relationships, generosity, love, and empathy but can be blocked by disappointments and pain. Its malfunction can lead to selfishness, isolation, inability to love, and diseases related to the heart and breath.

The fifth chakra
Vishuddha or throat chakra, is represented by the color blue and the element ether (space). It is located at the base of the throat and controls the neck, hands, and arms, and also listening and communication. It is blocked by lies, and its malfunction can cause problems related to the voice, vocal cords, thyroid malfunction, and fear of speaking to avoid problems.

The sixth chakra
Ajna or third eye chakra, is represented by the color blue and violet and the element of light. It is located in the center of the forehead and governs intuition, imagination, and mental clarity. This chakra is blocked by illusions, and its imbalance can lead to vision problems, migraines, mental confusion, and hallucinations.

The seventh chakra

Sahasrara or crown chakra, is related to the color purple or white and the element metal. It is located just above the head and controls the nervous system and the brain, but also wisdom and spirituality. An imbalance of it can lead to the need to manipulate and dominate others, to always wanting to be right, to bullying, and to mental rigidity. This chakra is important for connection with the spiritual dimension and a sense of unity with the universe.

Purify, Charge and Use crystals

Each crystal carries with it its own history, and it has the extraordinary ability to bind to any energy it has come into contact with, and being stones that can be millions of years old, it becomes essential to reset their charge and start anew. When we acquire new crystals, we must therefore prepare them with a cleansing so that we can make the most of their potential. The physical cleansing is then followed by the energetic cleansing that eliminates any negative vibrations that may have affected the crystal so as to zero out any accumulated energy.

Purify the stones

<u>Salt purification</u>: this treatment is the most aggressive of all, as it reprograms the crystal and erases all the information it has accumulated. The crystal should never come into direct contact with the salt as it may be damaged. It is recommended to place it in a small glass bowl that will be placed in a larger container containing water and salt. The glass allows an exchange of energy between the crystal and the salt, and in a couple of hours,

the stone will be purified.

Water purification: this method is effective for crystals that remain exposed in crowded environments and have direct contact with us. However, hot water can damage crystals, so it is recommended to use a shallow jet of cold water for a few minutes. Remember that not all crystals are compatible with water, so make sure this treatment is suitable for the stone you want to purify.

Clay purification: an excellent alternative to salt purification. Simply place the crystal in a small bag and soak it in green clay overnight. The same clay should not be reused to purify multiple stones because it becomes charged with negative energy.

Fumigation: this method was already used by American Indians and is still used today. It consists of burning a holy pole (a specific type of incense) or white sage and letting the smoke envelop the stone.

Purification with Bach flowers: this method involves pouring a few drops of Bach flower extract directly onto the crystal, leaving it for a few minutes, and rinsing it with running water. This method is not to be used with crystals that fear water.

Purification with earth: with this method, you purify and recharge the stone at the same time. Simply place the crystal wrapped in a cloth bag directly on the dry earth for five or six hours.

Recharge crystals and energize them

The next step after purification is crystal recharging, and it can be done in several ways:

Recharge with lunar energy: the crystal can be exposed to direct moonlight throughout the night. There are no particular contraindications.

Recharge with soil: ideally, the stones should be buried at the roots of a tree, but if your house does not allow it, the pot of your houseplant is ok. The stone can rest in the earth for a day or two.

Recharge with solar energy: you can expose the crystal to sunlight throughout the day, but avoid doing so with light-colored crystals such as quartz, which can change color and impair the stone's properties.

Recharge with the pyramid: If you have a miniature replica of the Cheops pyramid, place the crystal at its base for 24 hours.

Charging with snow: placing the crystal on snow will amplify lunar or solar energy.

<u>Recharge with other crystals</u>: the simplest and most effective method of recharging crystals is to place them amidst other crystals on top of a cluster (a set of cluster-shaped minerals characterized by many spikes protruding from the base) or a druse (a whole mass of many small crystals that can be formed from different minerals) overnight.

Finally, to thoughtfully store the crystal, you just have to make sure to store it in the light and near other stones; absolutely avoid drawers or dark places.

How to use crystals

Crystals can be used as jewelry: The most common use of crystals is as bracelets, necklaces, rings, and pendants to be worn. This was the earliest use of crystals, which were considered talismans that contained magical power capable of warding off bad luck and encouraging good fortune. Although crystals became popular as jewelry, in the past, they were also used as personal amulets to be kept with you at all times. Ancient shamans, for example, inserted small crystal shards under the skin to internalize their properties. Meditating with crystals is a way to explore our inner world. Crystals are a source of inspiration for meditation, and they can be placed near us during practice. After centering one's attention on breathing, one observes the crystal carefully, noting every detail of its shape, color, and texture.

One tries to grasp the inner essence of the crystal without identifying with it. Listening in a nonjudgmental and detached way can lead to the discovery of parts of ourselves that require attention.

Guide to crystals

Aquamarine..32
Agata...34
Amazonite..36
Amber...38
Amethyst..40
Green aventurine..42
Carnelian..44
Diamond...46
Diaspro...48
Hematite..50
Fluorite...52
Fuchsite...54
Jade...56

Garnet..58
Howlite..60
Labradorite..62
Lapislazuli..64
Larimar...66
Magnetite..68
Malachite...70
Moldavite...72
Tiger's eye..74
Onyx..76
Fire opal..78
Obsidian snowflake..80
Moonstone...82
Citrine quartz..84
Smoked quartz..86
Rose quartz..88
Rhodochrosite...90
Rubin...92
Selenite...94
Emerald...96
Sodalite...98
Tanzanite..100
Topaz...102
Green tourmaline..104
Turquoise..106
Sapphire..108
Zircon...110

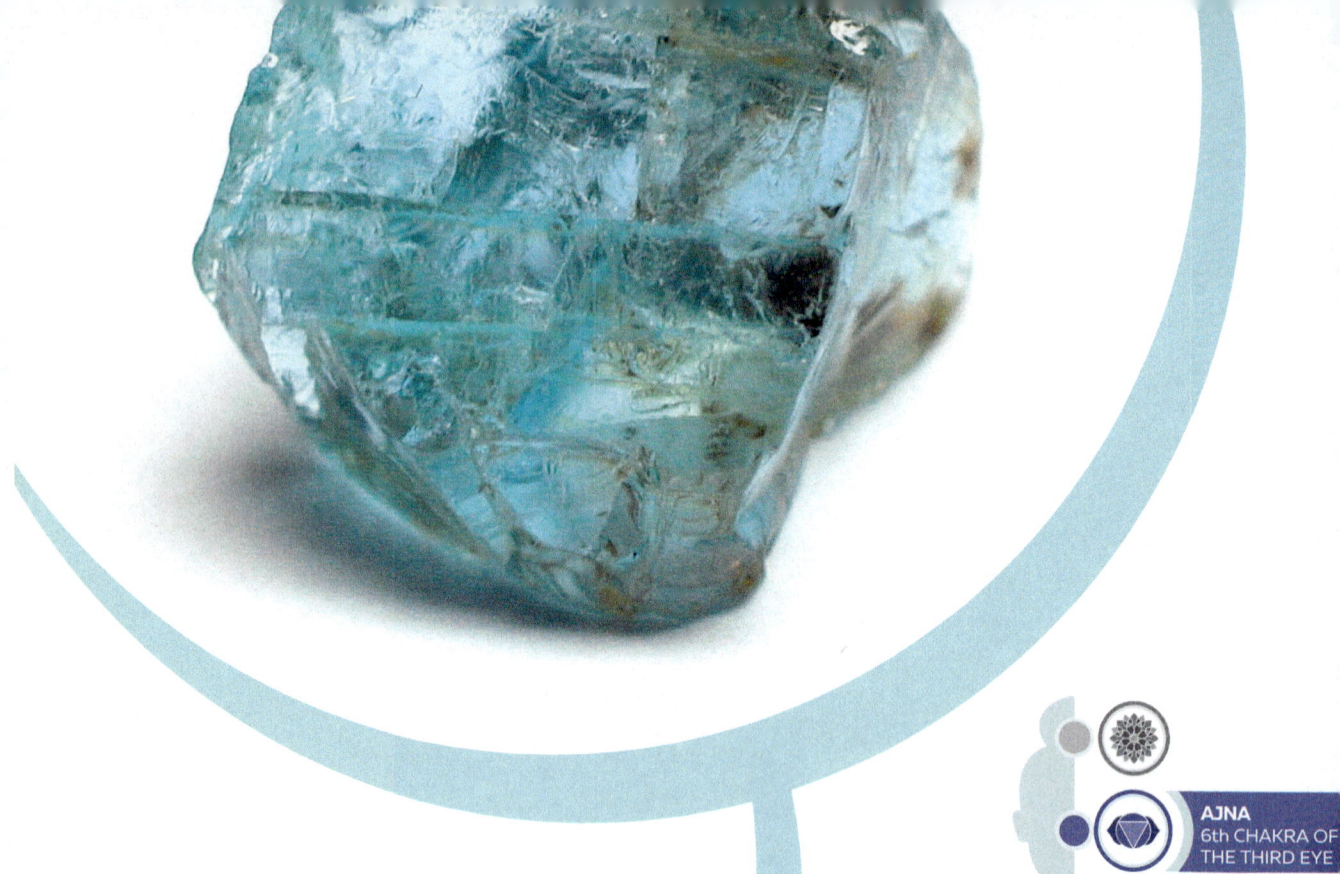

Aquamarine

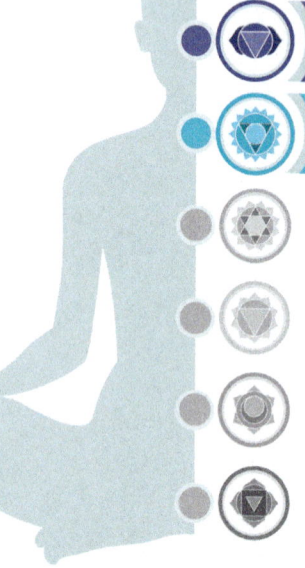

AJNA
6th CHAKRA OF THE THIRD EYE

VISHUDDHA
5th THROAT CHAKRA

Colors:
Green, Blue

Crystal structure:
Hexagonal

Zodiac sign:
Gemini, Libra, Aquarius, Pisces

History:
It is the stone of the goddess of the sea, so always used by sailors as an amulet to protect them during their sea voyages. These amulets were often thrown into the sea to appease Poseidon, the god of the seas.

Properties:
It promotes introspection, helps with mental clarity, and dissolves shyness. It is a stone that promotes peace and joy in relationships and allows us to express our thoughts peacefully.

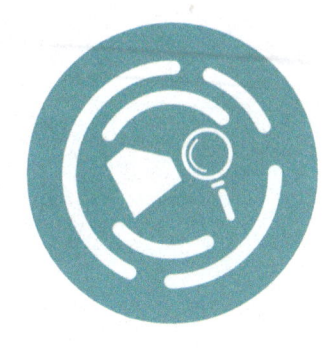

Body benefits:
Indicated for respiratory tract diseases and soothes throat diseases. Also used for inflammation of the gums and teeth.

Mind and spirit benefits:
It instills confidence, makes one sincere, and gives a sense of tranquility. Placing aquamarine near the heart while sleeping promotes restful sleep.

How to treat the stone:
Running water, or incense, is sufficient for purification. You can charge it with an amethyst druse or expose it to the Moon's rays.

Agata

VISHUDDHA
5th THROAT CHAKRA

ANAHATA
4th CHAKRA OF THE HEART

SVADHISHTHANA
2nd SPLENIC CHAKRA

MULADHARA
1st ROOT CHAKRA

Colors:
Lots of colors, muted and banded

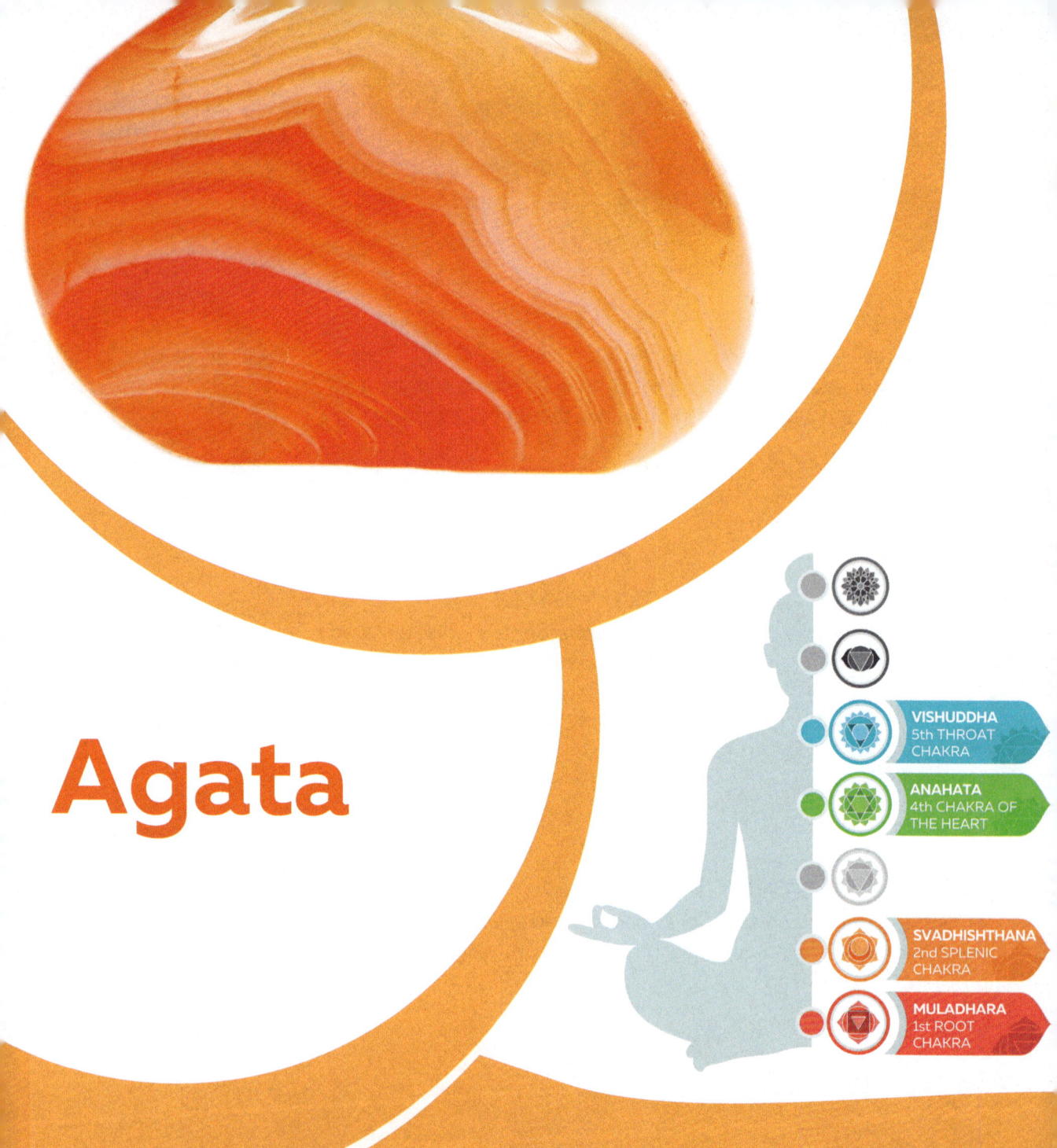

Crystal structure:
Trigonal

Zodiac sign:
Aries, Taurus, Scorpio

History:
Agate was once dissolved in water to counteract snake venom. In addition, it was a common belief that the person who wore agate as jewelry was well-regarded by God.

Properties:
Indicated in pregnancy to protect the fetus.

Body benefits:
Worn, helps improve concentration and perform self-analysis. Combined with lapis lazuli, it helps relieve insect bites.

Mind and spirit benefits:
Suitable for taking along on journeys, helps to recognize real desires.

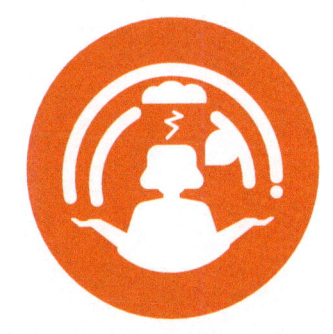

How to treat the stone:
Clean it with simple lukewarm water.

Amazonite

VISHUDDHA
5th THROAT CHAKRA

Colors:
Green, Blue

Crystal structure:
Triclinic

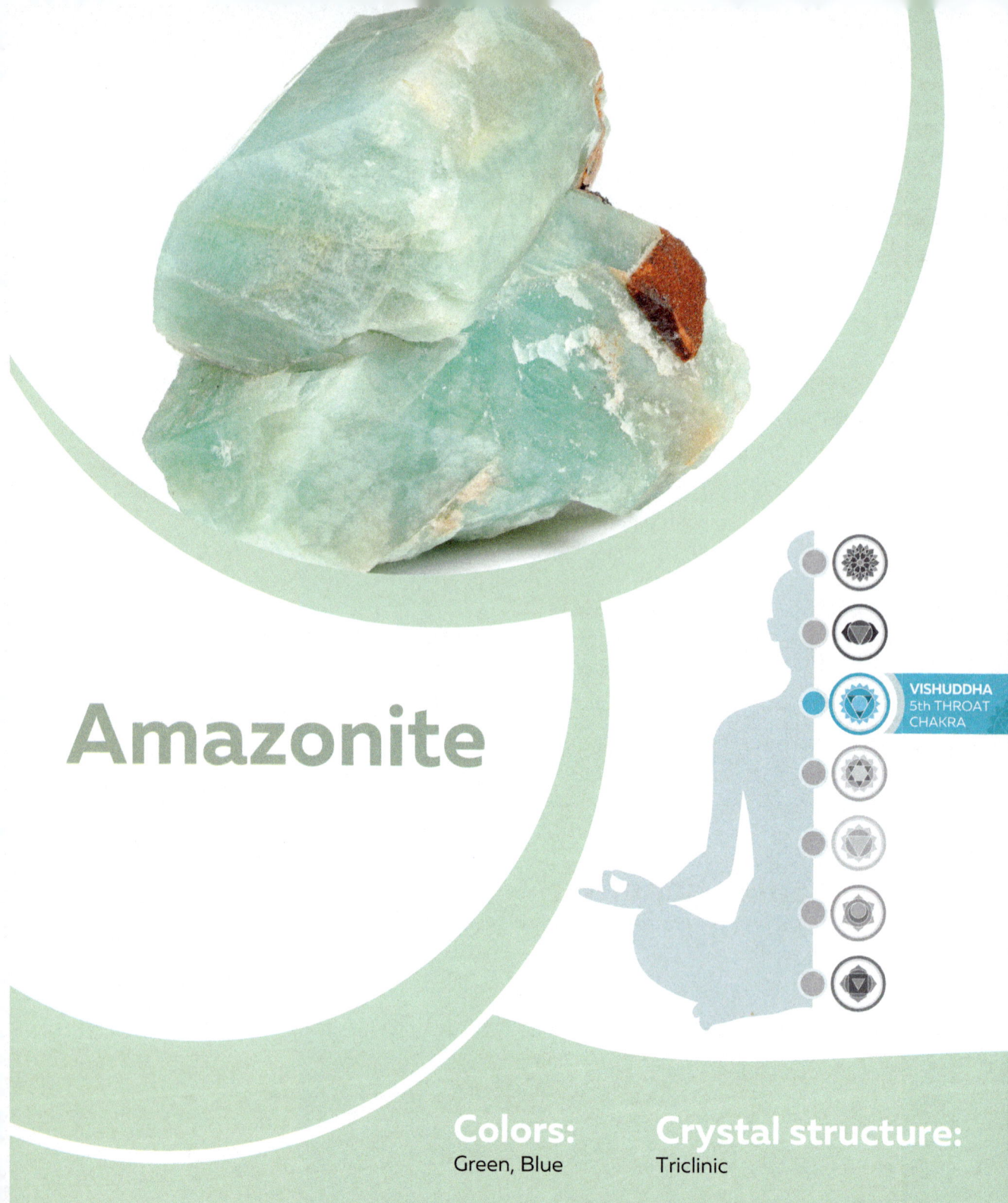

Zodiac sign:
Pisces, Virgo

History:
Amazonite is linked to the Amazon because of the intense turquoise that colors it and the peace it instills.

Properties:
Infuses positivity and love in communication with others; this stone makes us discover the gifts hidden within us.

Body benefits:
Most useful for preventing skin-related infections as it stimulates cellular reformation. Used as a necklace, we take advantage of the benefits related to the throat chakra; clasped between the hands, it helps to calm anxiety.

Mind and spirit benefits:
Increases resourcefulness and decision-making, brings back calm, and increases inner knowing. Absorbs radiation from computers and electronic devices.

How to treat the stone:
Purify it through fumigation with real incense.

Amber

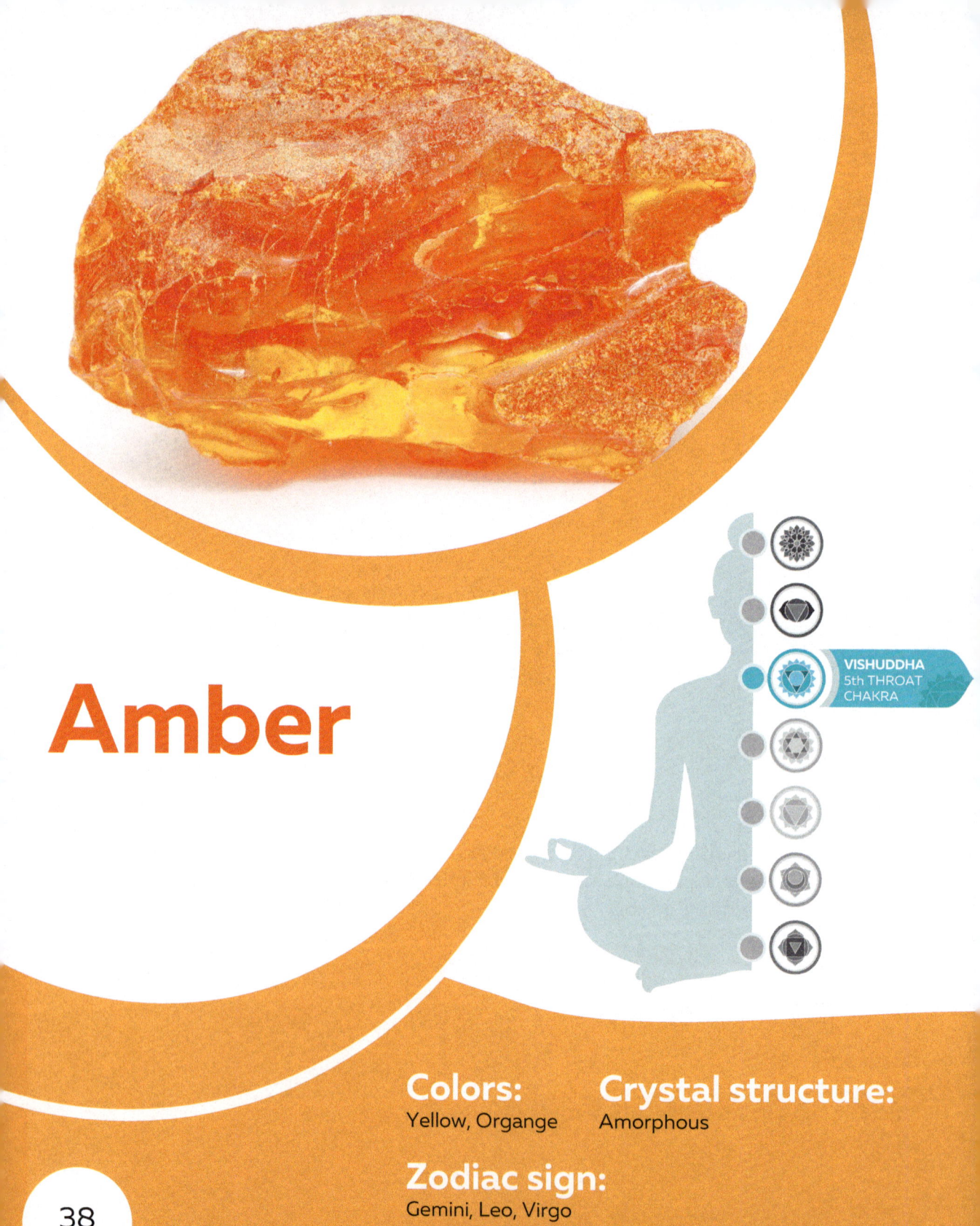

Colors:
Yellow, Organge

Crystal structure:
Amorphous

Zodiac sign:
Gemini, Leo, Virgo

VISHUDDHA
5th THROAT CHAKRA

History:
In ancient times, amber was used by hunters as a good-luck amulet because of its electrostatic ability, which was thought to attract what was desired.

Properties:
Brings optimism to the wearer and works on anxiety and depression.

Body benefits:
Helps manage certain types of pain, such as muscle tension at the stomach level, rheumatism, and arthritis, by strengthening all the joints in our body.

Mind and spirit benefits:
It helps us deal with the most stressful situations and is indicated to put things in perspective.

How to treat the stone:
To purify it, we can use the holy pole, clay that absorbs negative energies, earth, or contact with an amethyst druse.

Amethyst

SAHASRARA
7th CROWN CHAKRA

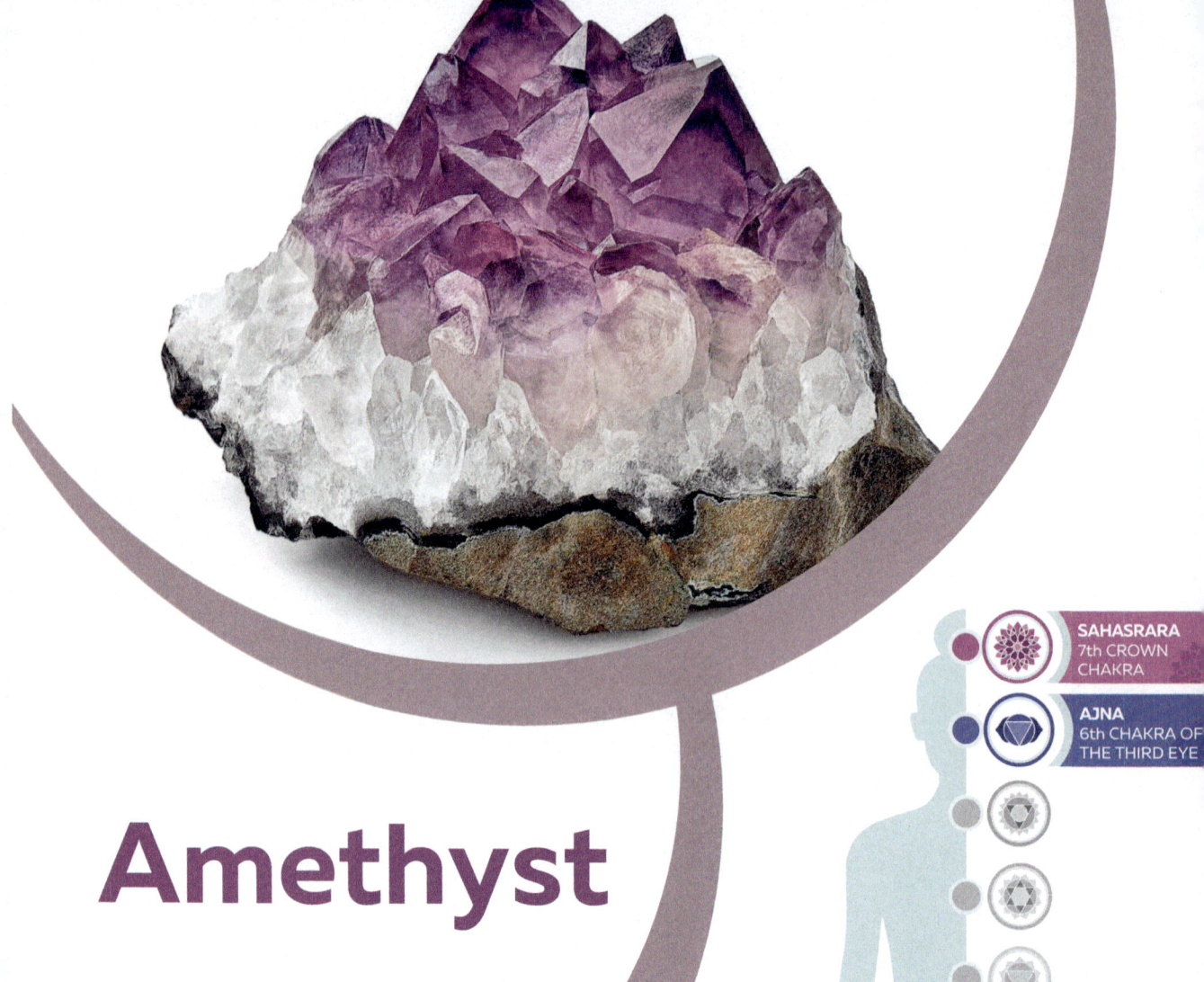

AJNA
6th CHAKRA OF THE THIRD EYE

Colors:
Purple

Crystal structure:
Trigonal

Zodiac sign:
Virgo, Pisces, Sagittarius

40

History:
Amethystos means one who does not get drunk, and it was believed that putting an amethyst crystal in a glass containing alcohol prevented the person from getting drunk. Legend has it that Amethyst is the name of a nymph who, fleeing from Bacchus, invoked Diana, who succeeded in transforming her into a crystal. The color purple, on the other hand, is attributed to her by Bacchus himself who, enraged, threw the chalice full of wine onto the stone.

Properties:
Developing awareness and scaling problems.

Body benefits:
Fights migraine and acts on the nervous system in general.

Mind and spirit benefits:
Placed under the pillow combats insomnia and placed on the ear combats tinnitus. Useful for meditation.

How to treat the stone:
It is charged with the rays of the sun and Moon and can be purified with water.

Green aventurine

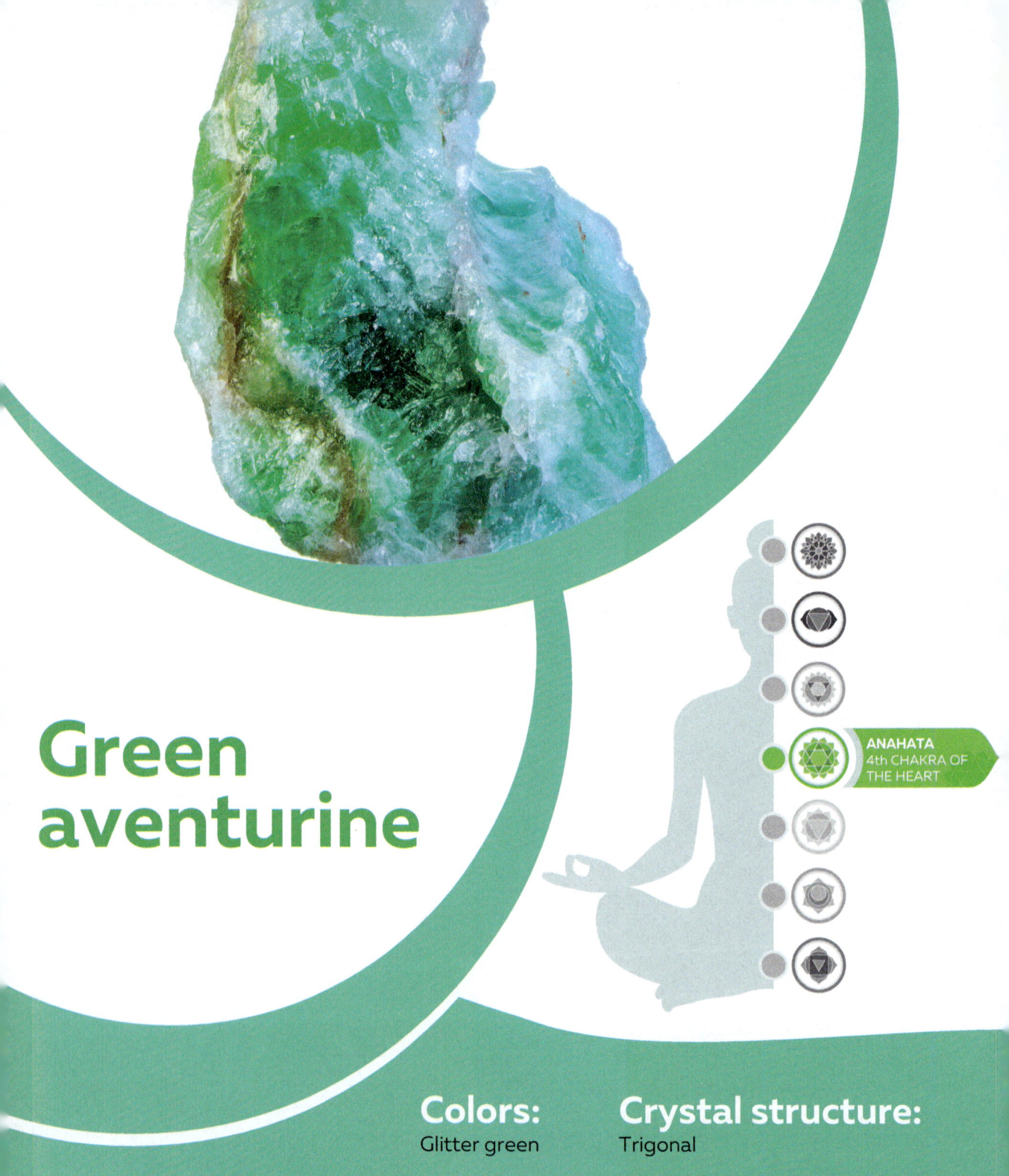

Colors:
Glitter green

Crystal structure:
Trigonal

Zodiac sign:
Taurus, Cancer

ANAHATA
4th CHAKRA OF THE HEART

History:
In Tibet, it was used to decorate statues that we can still admire today and was rumored to cure myopia; placed on statues, it symbolically displayed its visionary powers.

Properties:
Protects our vulnerability, gives us the confidence to take risks, and allows us to connect with our inner selves.

Body benefits:
Enhances visual faculties and regenerates the heart.

Mind and spirit benefits:
Helps us believe in ourselves and trust others, infuses the environment with a strong sense of security. Combined with other stones (turquoise, fire opal, or moonstone), it enables us to empathize with other people.

How to treat the stone:
Purify it with running water. To charge it, you can soak it in coarse salt or in contact with the earth.

Carnelian

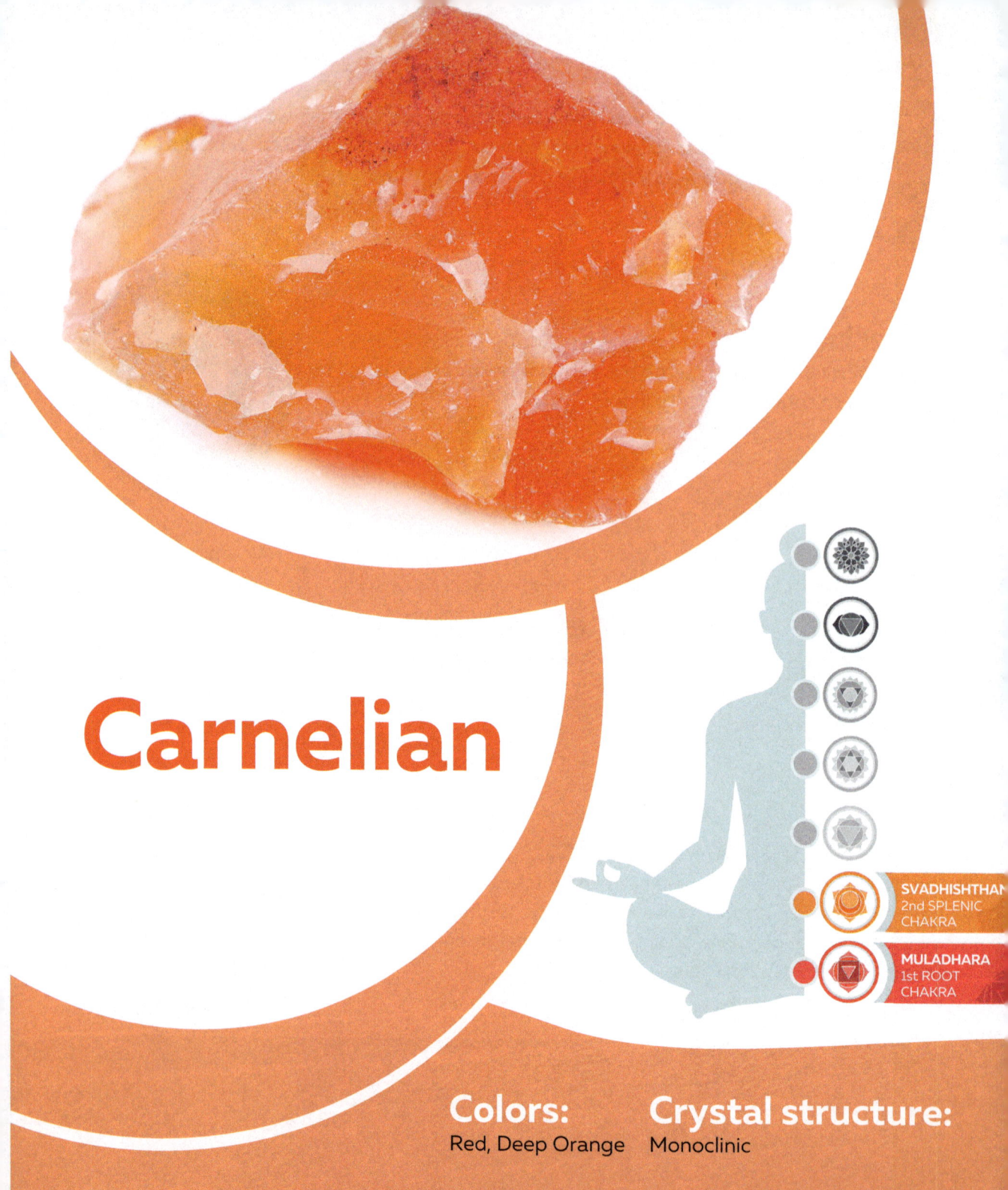

SVADHISHTHANA
2nd SPLENIC CHAKRA

MULADHARA
1st ROOT CHAKRA

Colors:
Red, Deep Orange

Crystal structure:
Monoclinic

Zodiac sign:
Aries, Virgo, Scorpio

History:
For the Egyptians, carnelian was the symbol of life because of its red color. It was called the "stone of the setting sun" and was placed on the deceased to accompany them on their journey to the afterlife; it is also featured on Tutankahmon's breastplate.

Properties:
It is a stone related to vitality and sexual energy and is a symbol of strength, determination, and courage.

Body benefits:
Effective for treating abdominal problems, helps liver and kidneys, promotes digestion, and regulates bowels. It also increases fertility.

Mind and spirit benefits:
Helps ward off negativity by improving mood and promoting optimism. Helps us not to be influenced by the judgments of others. Placed in the soil helps maintain its fertility.

How to treat the stone:
Purify it with incense. To charge it, we can leave it exposed to the Moon's rays or with an amethyst druse. Do not leave it exposed to the sun.

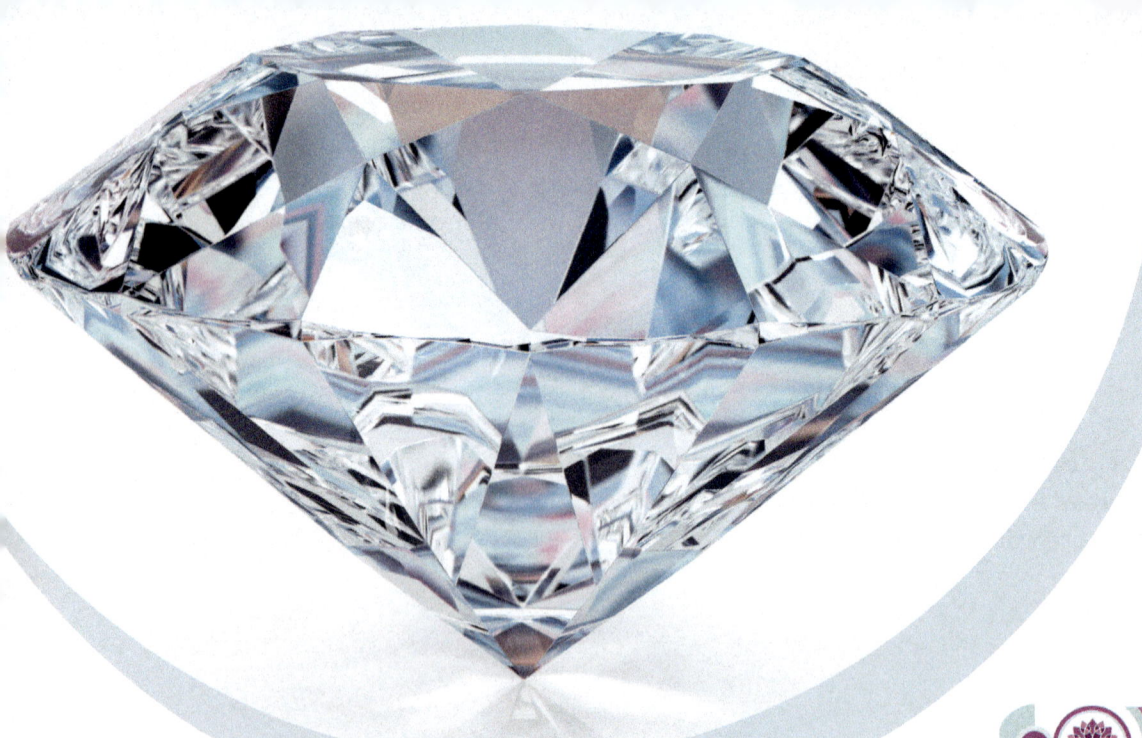

Diamond

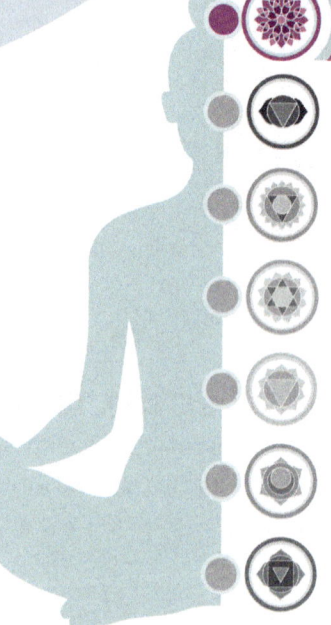

SAHASRARA
7th CROWN CHAKRA

Colors:
Transparent

Crystal structure:
Cubic

Zodiac sign:
Affine to all signs

History:
From the Greek, Adamas (unbreakable) has always been admired and revered by all peoples and religions. It is the strongest and most durable stone in nature, so it gives strength, purity, and innocence and amplifies emotions (both positive and negative). According to one legend, the diamond was created by a deity who decided to unite all the stones to form a very hard and clear one that holds them all within itself.

Properties:
The Stone of Unbreakable Promise is a symbol of eternal, faithful, and pure love. Useful if you are going through a period when you need to learn new concepts.

Body benefits:
It has the power to regenerate and purify and overcome fears and depressive states. Enhances our physical energy.

Mind and spirit benefits:
A diamond in the space instills feelings of joy, openness, and warmth.

How to treat the stone:
All methods except sunlight are fine for purifying the diamond. To charge it, we can leave it exposed to moonlight or use an amethyst druse.

Diaspro

Colors:
Brown, Black, Red

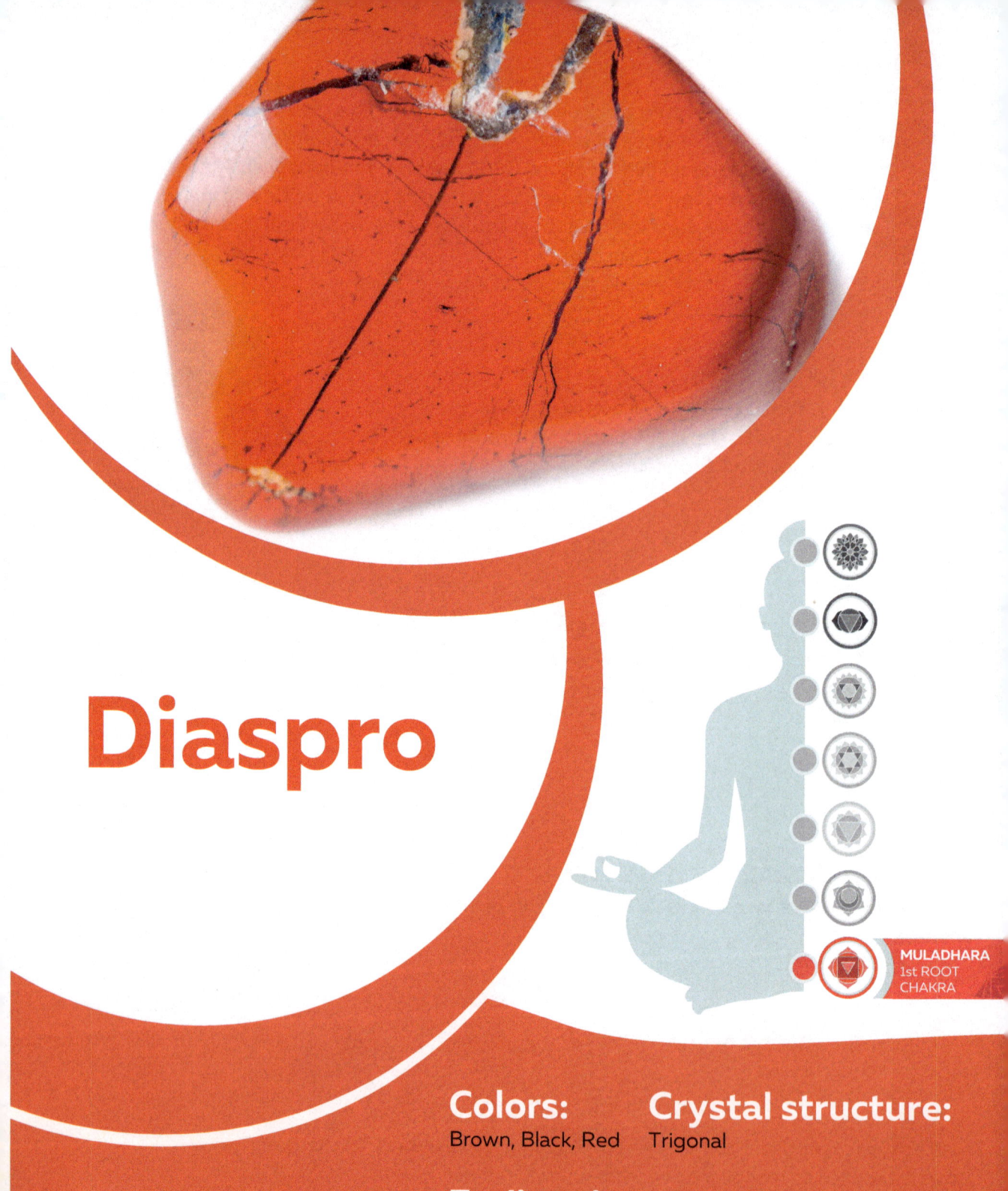

Crystal structure:
Trigonal

Zodiac sign:
Aries, Scorpio

MULADHARA
1st ROOT CHAKRA

48

History:
It was used by the Etruscans and Egyptians to remove spells and curses.

Properties:
Red jasper increases our decision-making power and helps us free ourselves from the emotional dependence of people.

Body benefits:
Helps oxygenate the blood, indicated for those with iron deficiency, and improves the immune system.

Mind and spirit benefits:
On a spiritual level, jasper can be used to eliminate prejudices and pursue individual goals so that the way forward becomes clearer.

How to treat the stone:
Purify it with clay, amethyst druse, or real incense. Charge it with sunlight.

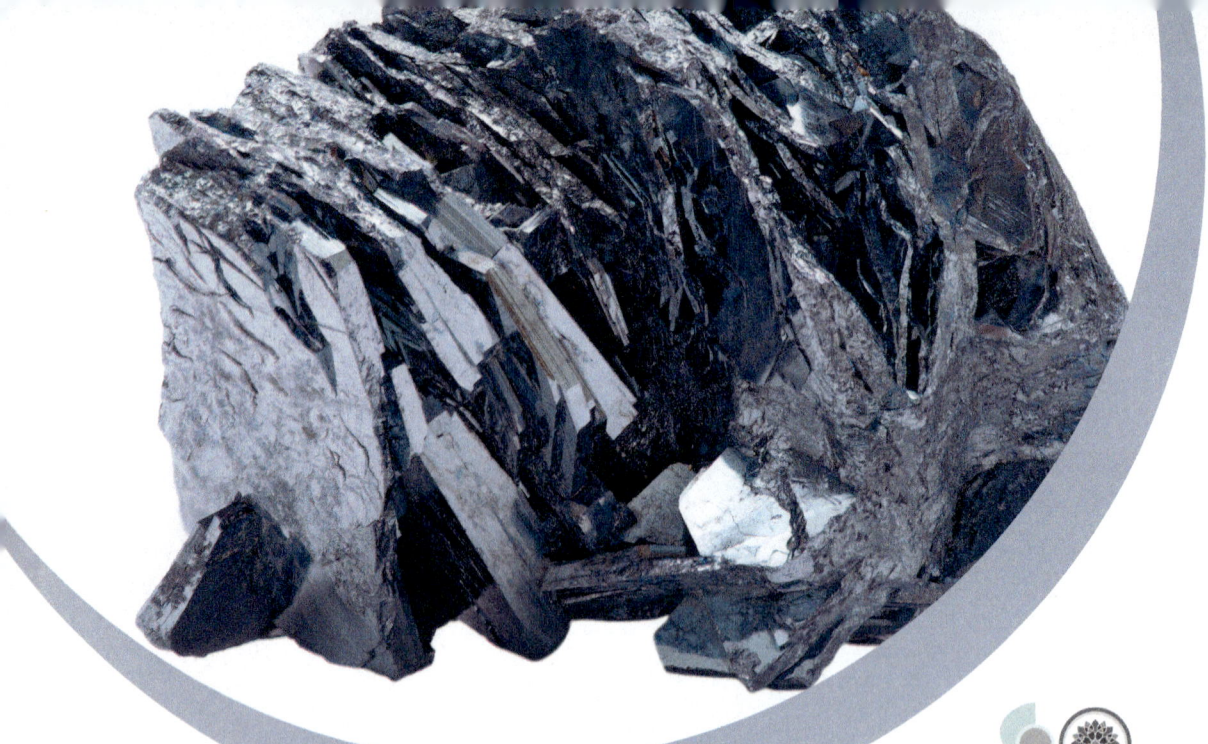

Hematite

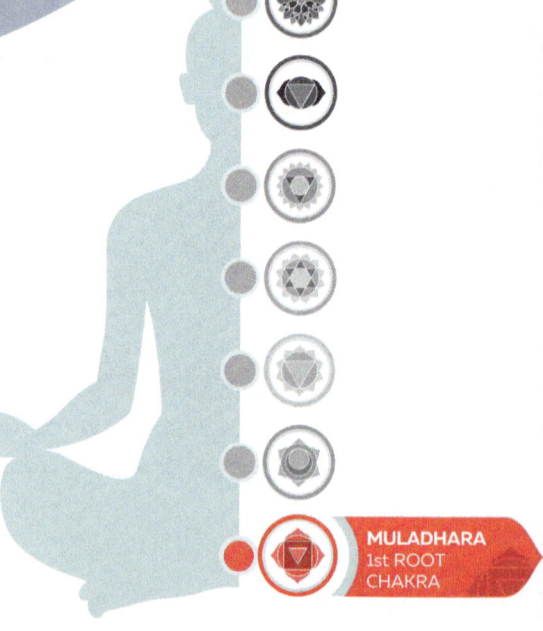

MULADHARA 1st ROOT CHAKRA

Colors:
Gray, Metallic black, Red

Crystal structure:
Trigonal

Zodiac sign:
Virgo, Scorpio

History:
Hematite is derived from Greek and means "bloodstone." It was used by the Egyptians and Babylonians to help heal wounds because of its power to accelerate blood production and speed up blood clotting. This is why it was put on the wounded in war and was, therefore, always stained with blood, hence its name.

Properties:
This stone creates a real protective shield around the wearer so as to prevent contamination by negativity. It stimulates the will and imparts dynamism.

Body benefits:
Helps produce red blood cells and improves iron assimilation by the intestines, useful in cases of anemia.

Mind and spirit benefits:
Most suitable for those who are impulsive and distracted by nature but also for those who are very susceptible to criticism and comments from others.

How to treat the stone:
It can be purified with water, and you can charge it through the energy of the Moon's rays.

Fluorite

AJNA
6th CHAKRA OF THE THIRD EYE

Colors:
Yellow, Green, Blue, Purple

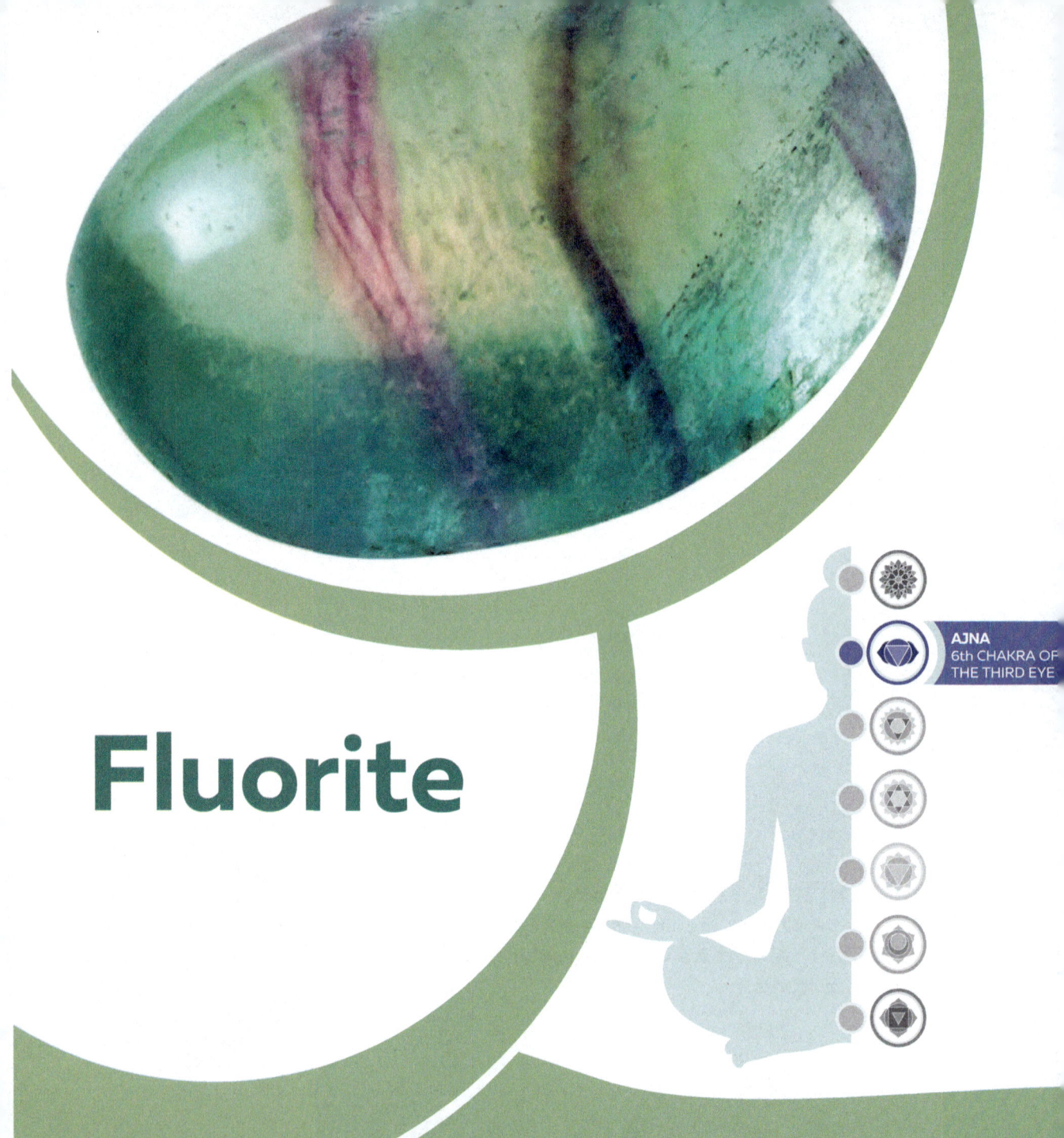

Crystal structure:
Cubic

Zodiac sign:
Taurus, Aries, Leo, Scorpio

52

History:
When exposed to ultraviolet light, it exhibits the fluorescence effect, hence its name. In ancient times it was considered used as a substitute for precious stones in jewelry making. It is also referred to as the "Genius Stone" because of its mind-elevating characteristic.

Properties:
Promotes free thinking, helps us not to be influenced by others, and to seek our own autonomy by increasing our confidence.

Body benefits:
Helps regenerate lung tissue, promotes calcium absorption, then strengthens bones and teeth. Helps regulate body fluids.

Mind and spirit benefits:
Perfect for getting rid of physical and emotional addictions and restoring a balance between mind and heart. The Fluorite pyramid is perfect for meditation.

How to treat the stone:
Purify it with incense or running water. It is a very delicate stone, so treat it with care.

Fuchsite

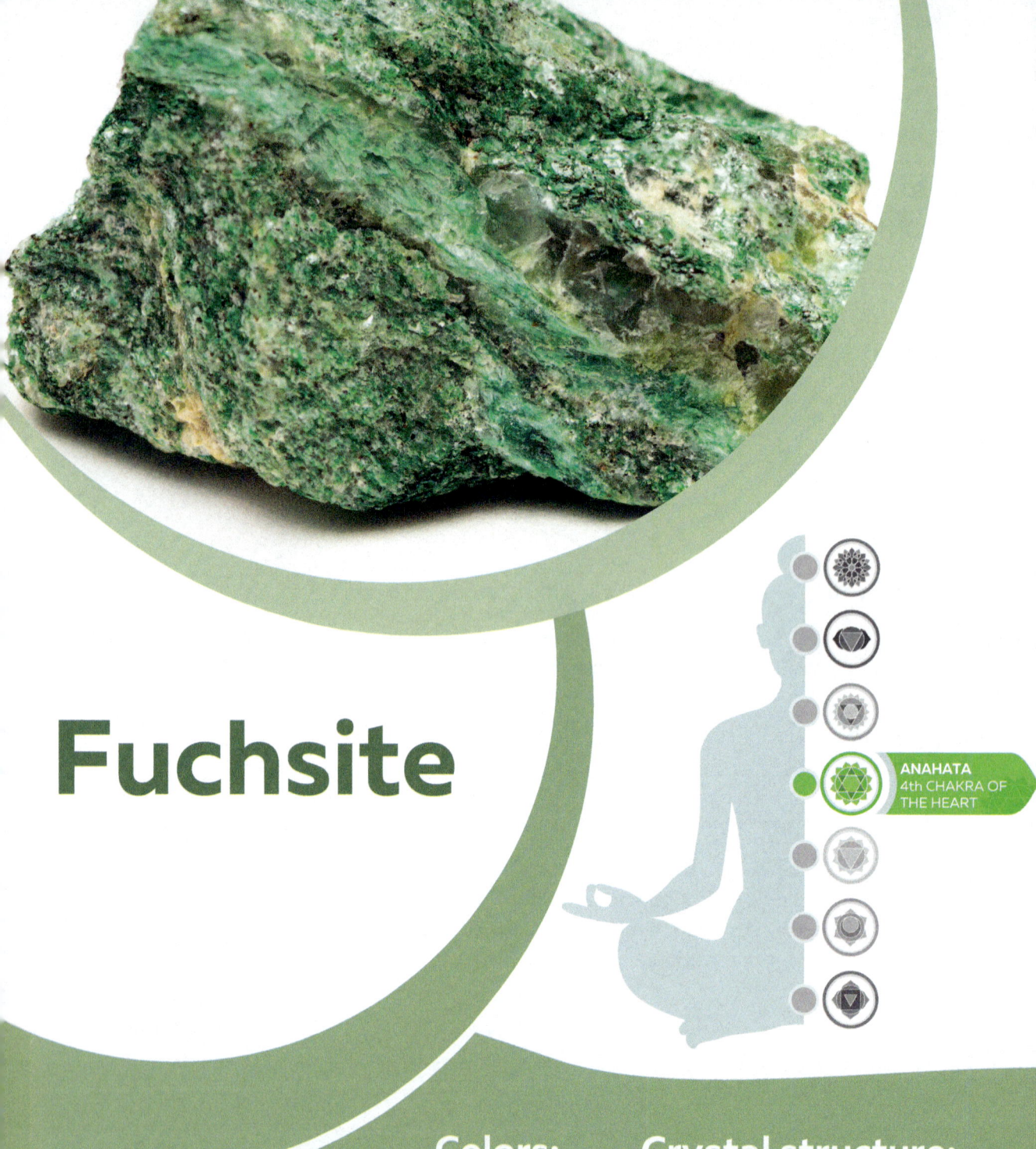

Colors:
Green

Crystal structure:
Monoclinic

Zodiac sign:
Acquarius

ANAHATA
4th CHAKRA OF THE HEART

54

History:
The stone is named after the mineralogist who discovered it, German mineralogist Johann von Fuchs.

Properties:
It helps to appreciate the little things and put everything in perspective. It attracts lightheartedness and compassion; it is the stone of renewal.

Body benefits:
Worn helps remove toxic substances from the body and helps heal burns, itching, and rashes. Useful to keep at home when there is a sick person because it has healing abilities.

Mind and spirit benefits:
It helps to cure insomnia, is a relaxing stone, and helps to handle problems with greater detachment.

How to treat the stone:
Do not immerse in water. It can be charged with a rock crystal or an amethyst.

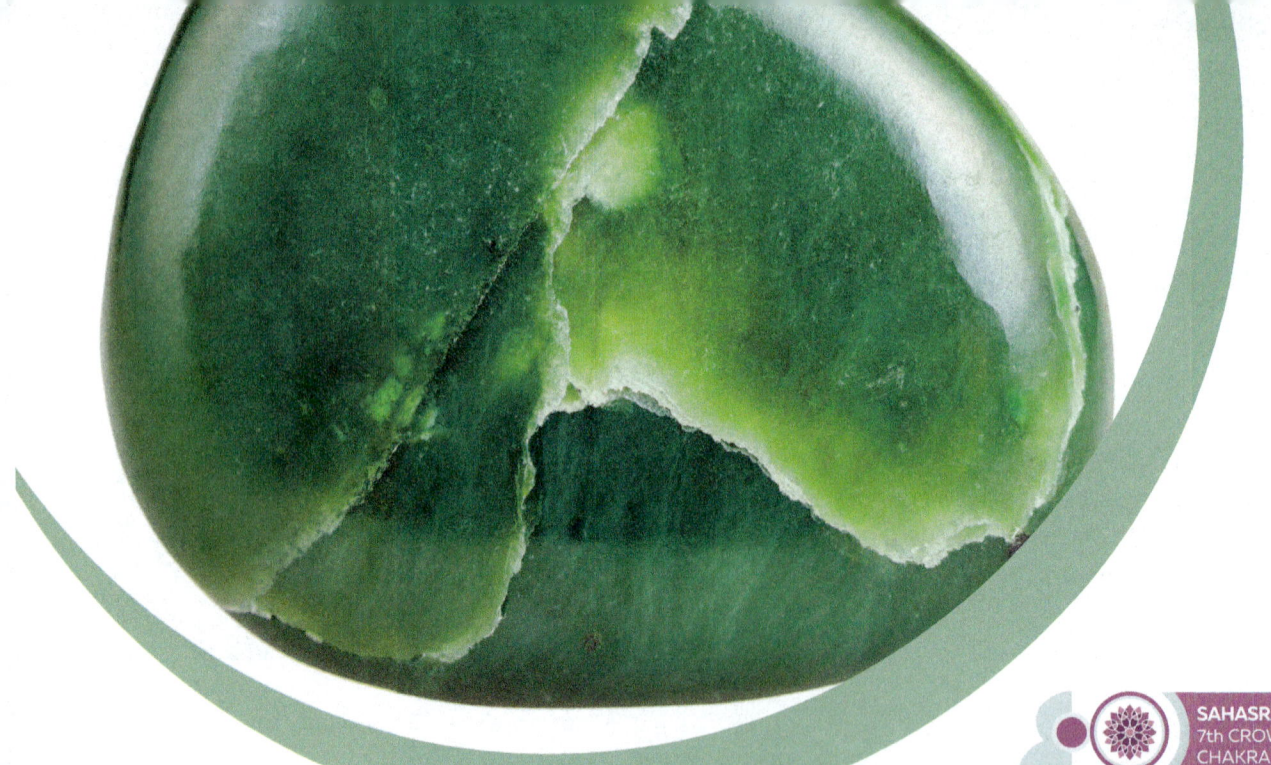

Jade

Colors:
Green, White, Yellow, Purple, Black, Red

Zodiac sign:
Cancer, Aquarius

Crystal structure:
Monoclinic

- SAHASRARA — 7th CROWN CHAKRA
- AJNA — 6th CHAKRA OF THE THIRD EYE
- VISHUDDHA — 5th THROAT CHAKRA
- ANAHATA — 4th CHAKRA OF THE HEART
- MANIPURA — 3rd SOLAR PLEXUS CHAKRA
- SVADHISHTHAN — 2nd SPLENIC CHAKRA
- MULADHARA — 1st ROOT CHAKRA

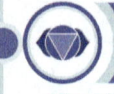

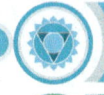

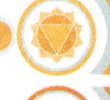

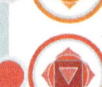

History:
It was defined by Confucius as "a mirror of soul-mind integrity," and he claimed that it had the power to make decisions with confidence and determination. In Eastern cultures, it was auspicious to give it as a gift at the birth of a child.

Properties:
Symbolizes long life and attracts good fortune, as well as helping us channel life force to evolve.

Body benefits:
Helps eliminate impurities in organs, restoring a state of well-being and improving bone joints. Helps decrease pain related to cramps.

Mind and spirit benefits:
It is a protective talisman, has calming properties and eliminates fear, and invites benevolence.

How to treat the stone:
Purify it with a holy pole or by placing it on an amethyst druse, but also with clay and earth. It should not be exposed to sunlight.

Garnet

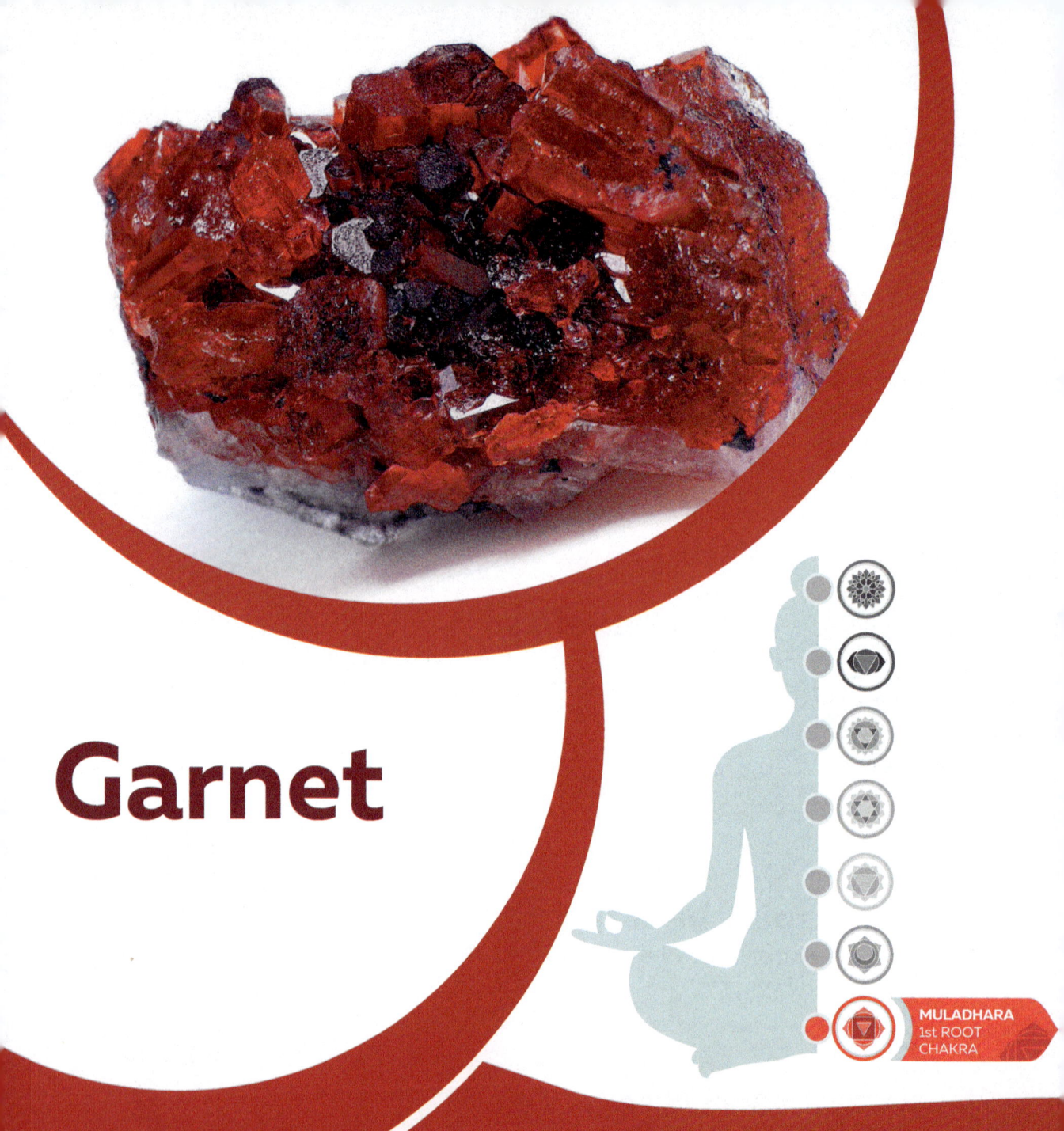

MULADHARA 1st ROOT CHAKRA

Colors:
Red

Crystal structure:
Cubic

Zodiac sign:
Aries, Taurus, Libra

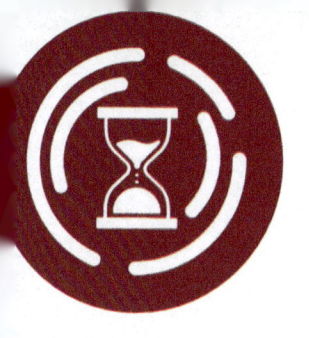

History:
The name garnet comes from granatum, meaning pomegranate, and is associated with the seeds of this autumn fruit because of its shape.

Properties:
If we need to change something on a spiritual level, we can use garnet to break the energies stagnating within us and become who we really desire. Garnet helps us form passions and attract libido, as it harnesses the energies of Venus, Aphrodite, and Cupid and makes us more confident in our sexual abilities.

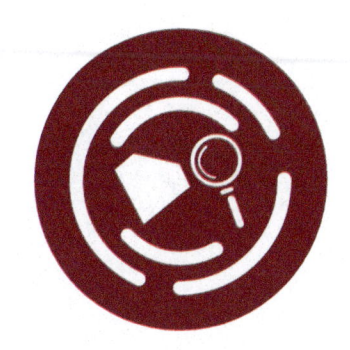

Body benefits:
Purifies our negative energies by eliminating excess waste and toxins, regulates blood pressure and internal rhythms specifically, but also identifies the reason why we want to eat a certain food or feel tired because it awakens the mind and makes us realize that it needs the body.

Mind and spirit benefits:
It revitalizes our body and balances our inner strength, and is helpful in figuring out which direction to take in life.

How to treat the stone:
To charge the garnet, we can simply place it under running water for three minutes or on rock crystals.

Howlite

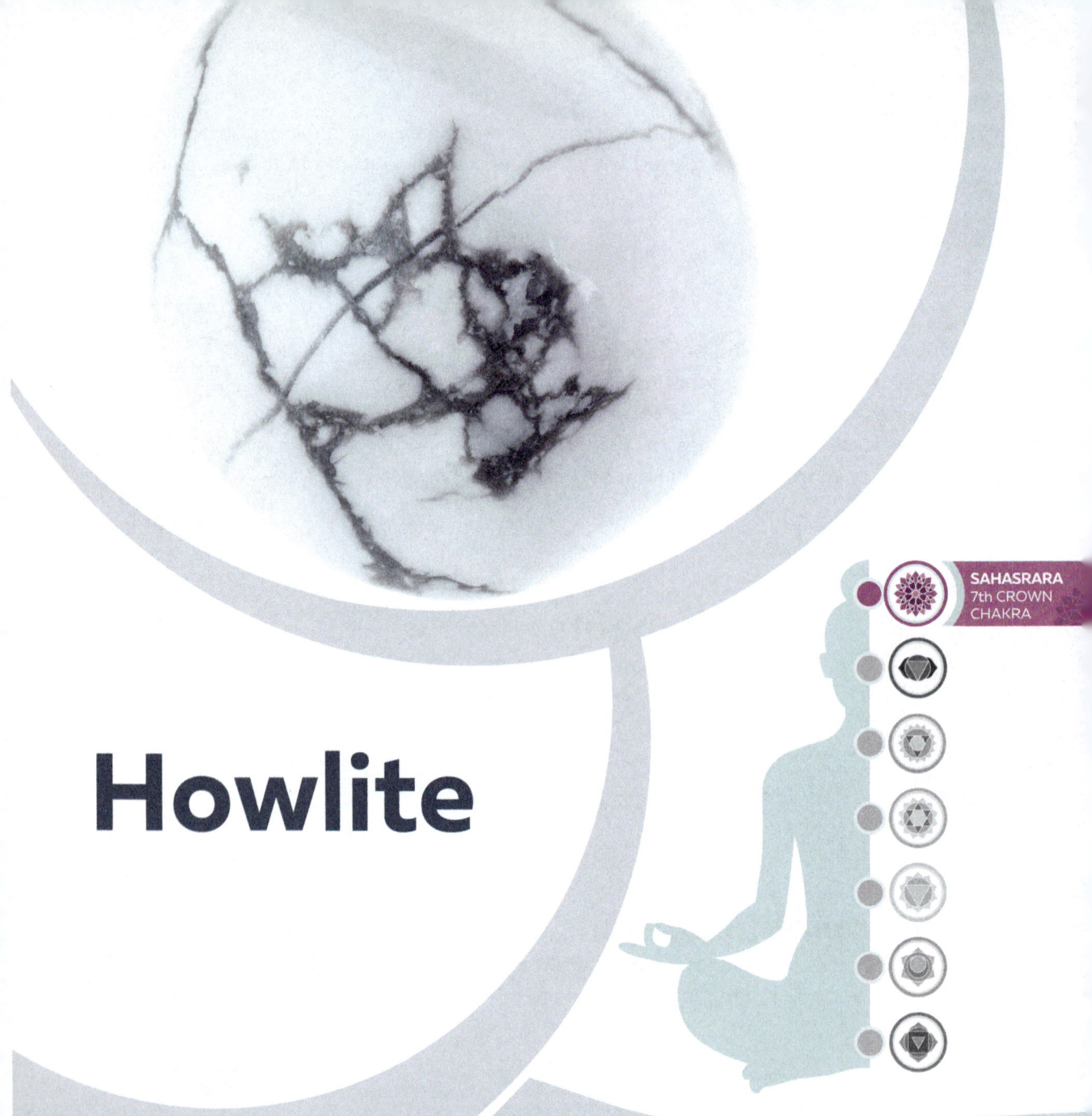

SAHASRARA
7th CROWN CHAKRA

Colors:
White with gray veins

Crystal structure:
Monoclinic

Zodiac sign:
Cancer, Sagittarius, Aquarius

History:
It was discovered only recently by Canadian chemist Henri How, and after his death, it was named after him.

Properties:
Helps heal wounds, overcome pain and metabolize anger.

Body benefits:
Helps treat insomnia and can be a good ally in preventing cramps. Helps improve blood oxygenation. Recommended during diets because it has a diuretic effect and prevents water retention.

Mind and spirit benefits:
Helps maintain self-control, gives calm, and prevents us from impulsive reactions. Used in cases of anxiety, shock, and panic. Placed in the center of the room allows us to create a healthy relationship with our surroundings.

How to treat the stone:
To charge it, we can leave it exposed to the sun's rays or with a quartz druse. Running water instead to purify it.

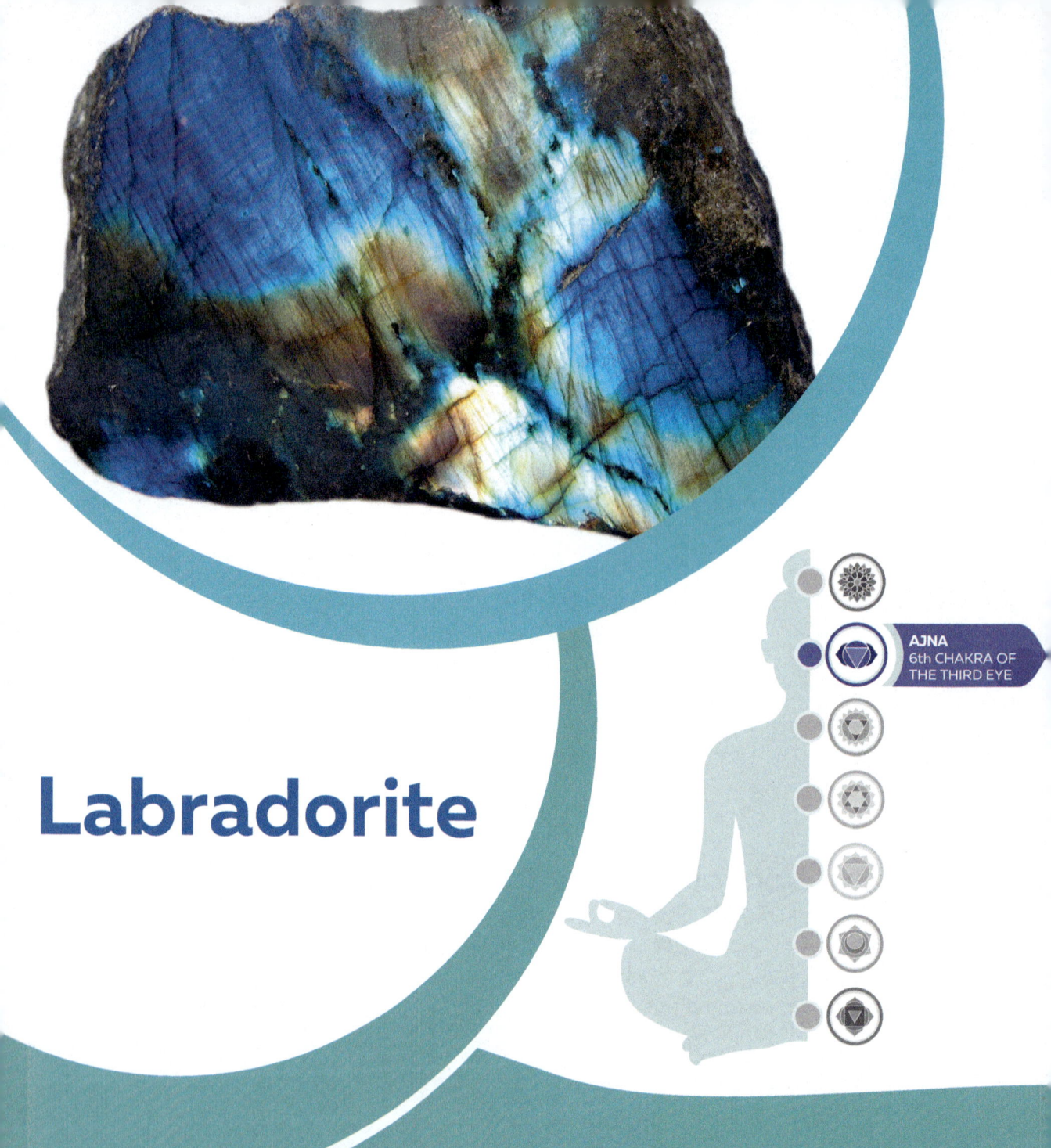

Labradorite

AJNA
6th CHAKRA OF THE THIRD EYE

Colors:
Blue

Crystal structure:
Triclinic

Zodiac sign:
Pisces, Cancer, Sagittarius

History:
Discovered on the Labrador Peninsula in Canada. According to the Inuit, the people who live straddling Greenland, Canada, and the United States, labradorite is said to be a frozen fire that fell to Earth from the aurora borealis. This is because of its extraordinary color that reflects that enchanted and magical light.

Properties:
This stone is prized for its metallic reflections and magical properties. All over the world, it is used by shamans and those in search of lucid dreams, the oneironauts.

Body benefits:
This stone helps us awaken our mental abilities, also going to stimulate our imagination. It allows us to get in touch with spirit guides.

Mind and spirit benefits:
Labradorite helps us overcome depression caused by our inability to relate to others or to cure addictions to smoking and alcohol.

How to treat the stone:
To charge it, we can take advantage of the energies of the Moon and absolutely avoid soaking it in water. To purify it, we can use incense fumigation or green clay.

Lapislazzuli

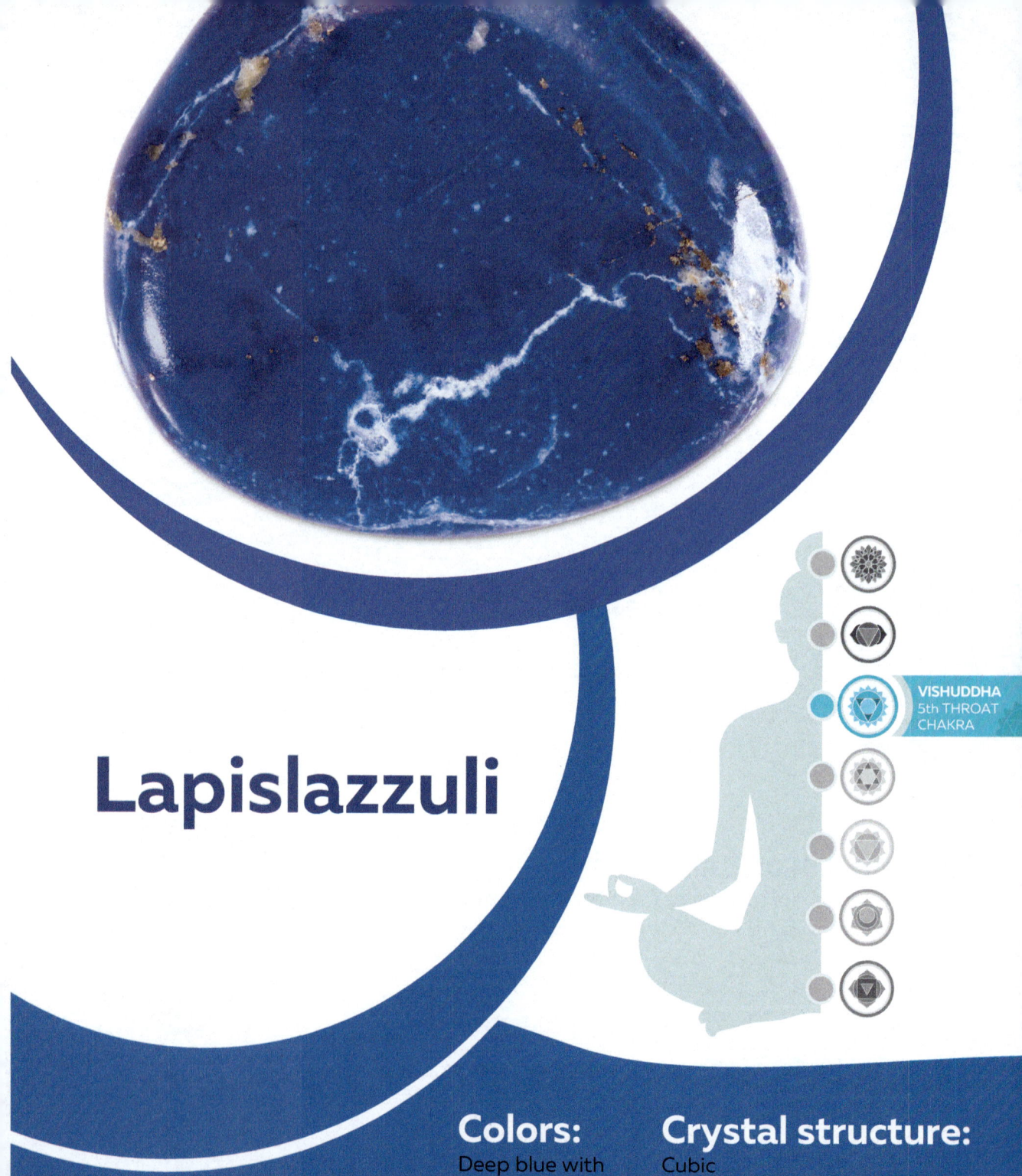

VISHUDDHA
5th THROAT CHAKRA

Colors:
Deep blue with gold veins

Crystal structure:
Cubic

Zodiac sign:
Aquarius, Pisces, Sagittarius

64

History:
According to the ancient Egyptians, lapis lazuli was one of the most important and sacred stones as it was used to make up a necklace worn by the High Priest and to create scarab-shaped seals. It was used to purify the souls of the deceased, and they pulverized it by mixing it with gold to create a paste that was then placed on the skull.

Properties:
Promotes reasoning, wisdom, and intellect, making us more curious and livelier.

Body benefits:
Worn as a necklace, it is ideal for those who seek their own expressiveness, for those who want to reduce anger, and for those who want to accept themselves for who they are.

Mind and spirit benefits:
This stone helps us work on dreams, grasping their meaning and making us more aware and intuitive.

How to treat the stone:
To charge this stone, we can use moonbeams, while to purify it, we can use incense or green clay, but also by placing the crystal on top of an amethyst druse.

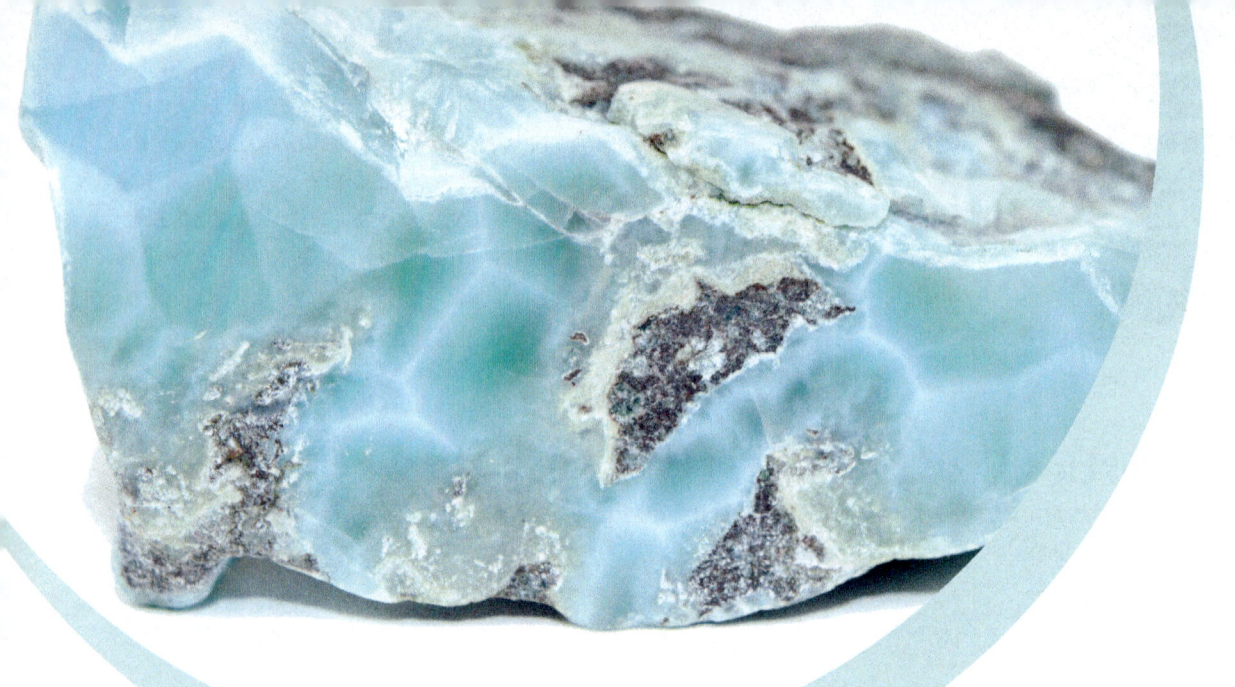

Larimar

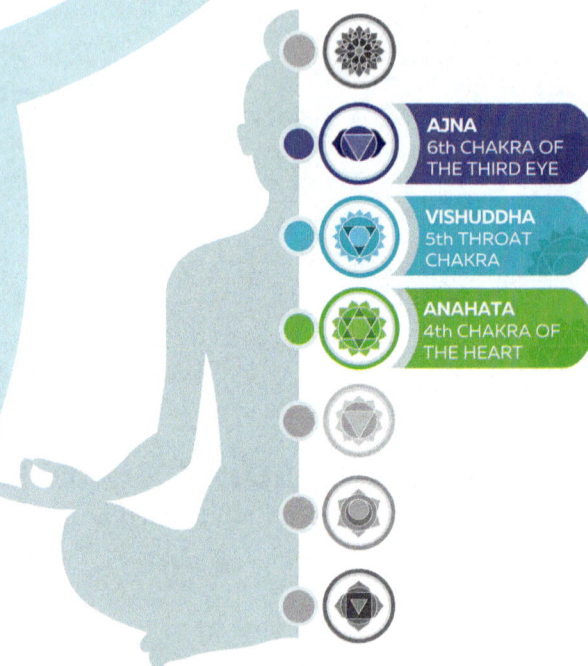

AJNA
6th CHAKRA OF THE THIRD EYE

VISHUDDHA
5th THROAT CHAKRA

ANAHATA
4th CHAKRA OF THE HEART

Colors:
Light Blue, Turquoise

Crystal structure:
Rhombic

Zodiac sign:
Leo, Pisces

History:
According to the Taino (people of the Dominican Republic), the sea stone, as it was named, had magical properties against negative energies and evil spirits and promoted communication with sea-related deities.

Properties:
It is used as a healing stone and helps reduce anxiety and stress and release emotional blocks.

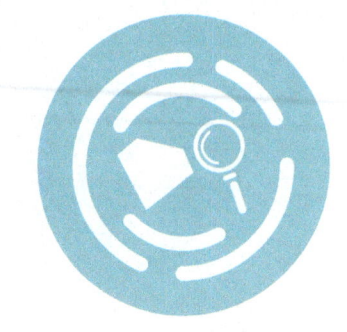

Body benefits:
It helps to improve our skin, strengthen the immune system, treat breathing-related problems such as bronchitis and asthma, and improve digestion and blood circulation.

Mind and spirit benefits:
Promotes meditation and keeps negative energies away. Placed in the home or workplace ensures a pleasant atmosphere.

How to treat the stone:
To clean the Larimar, we can use a dry and soft cloth, avoiding too high temperatures and chemicals that are aggressive and could ruin it.

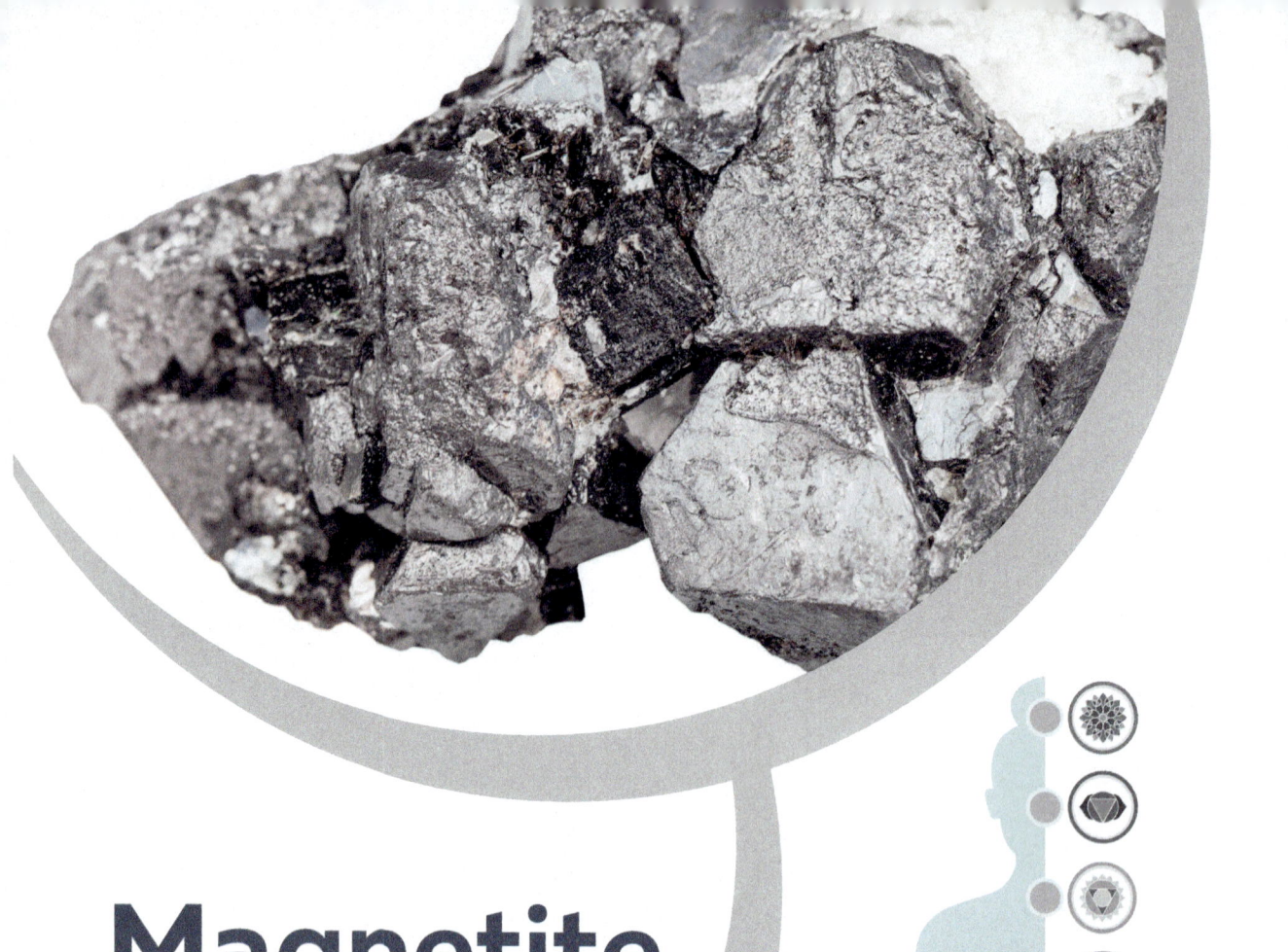

Magnetite

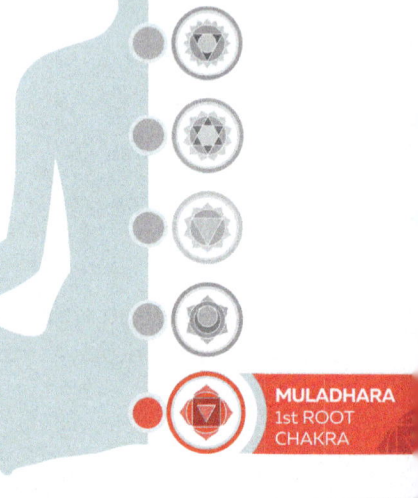

Colors:
Black

Crystal structure:
Cubic

Zodiac sign:
Aries, Capricorn

MULADHARA
1st ROOT CHAKRA

History:
For so many years, this stone has been used for its magnetic properties; in fact, the compass was created precisely because of its physical properties.

Properties:
Magnetite relieves tension and boosts sexual energy.

Body benefits:
Due to its magnetic properties, it is useful for our health by acting as a natural anti-inflammatory.

Mind and spirit benefits:
Its power of attraction ensures that it is able to capture negative energies from the environment and body and then disperse them into the cosmos.

How to treat the stone:
To charge the magnetite, simply expose it to sunlight.

Malachite

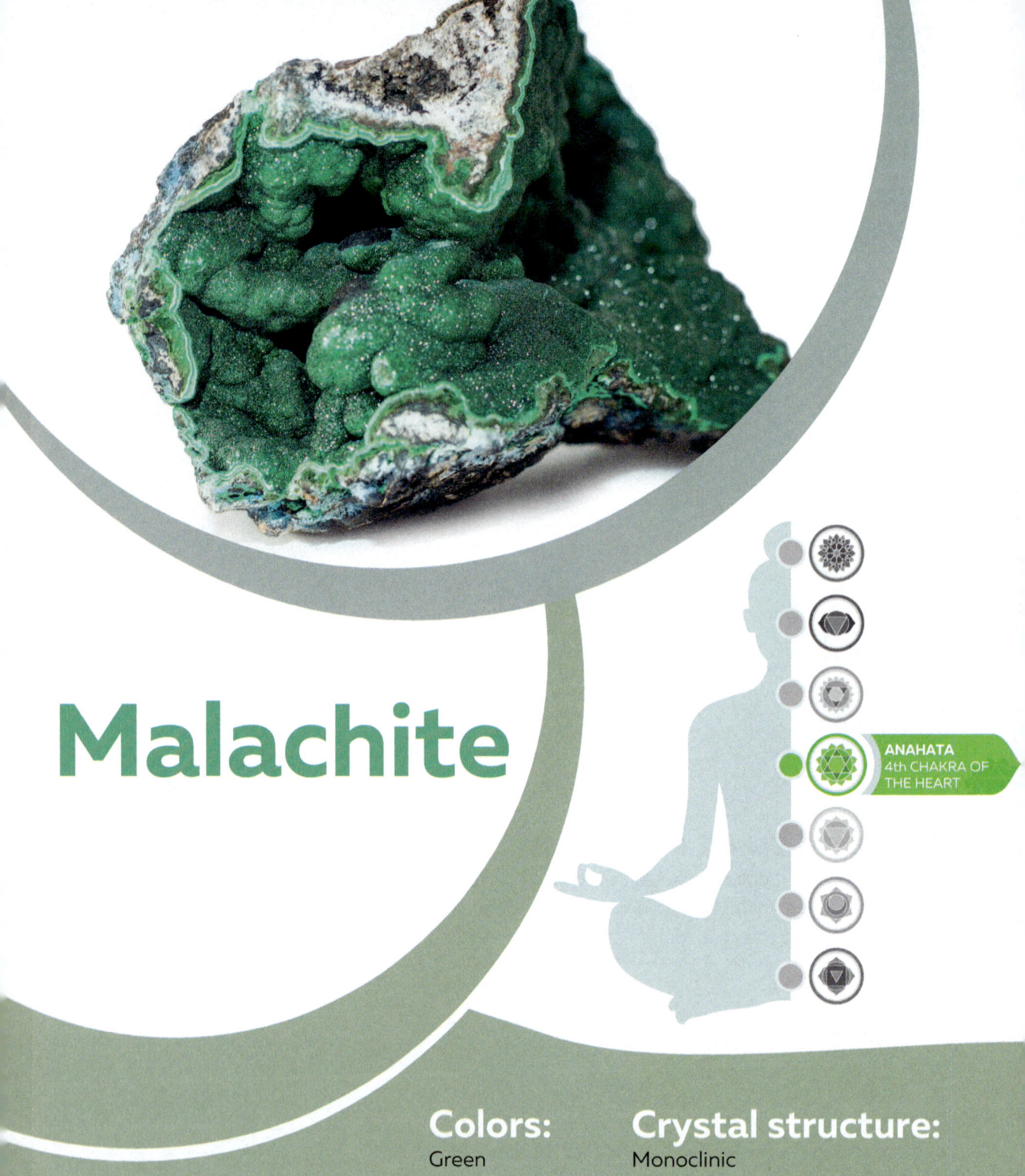

Colors:
Green

Crystal structure:
Monoclinic

Zodiac sign:
Libra, Taurus, Capricorn

ANAHATA
4th CHAKRA OF THE HEART

History:
Always sacred to a female deity, such as Persephone or Isis, it was used to protect children from evil spirits and was attached to the very cradle of the newborn to promote peaceful dreams.

Properties:
Makes one sharper in observing details and critical thinking skills.

Body benefits:
Regulates the menstrual cycle and is recommended for memory problems, as well as having anti-inflammatory properties. Ideal against motion sickness.

Mind and spirit benefits:
It supports us during our inner evolution and roots us well to the ground, balancing our feelings and giving us awareness of their fluidity. Absorbs electromagnetic radiation and negative energies.

How to treat the stone:
Purify with incense, or with fresh water, or quartz druse.

Moldavite

SAHASRARA
7th CROWN CHAKRA

AJNA
6th CHAKRA OF THE THIRD EYE

ANAHATA
4th CHAKRA OF THE HEART

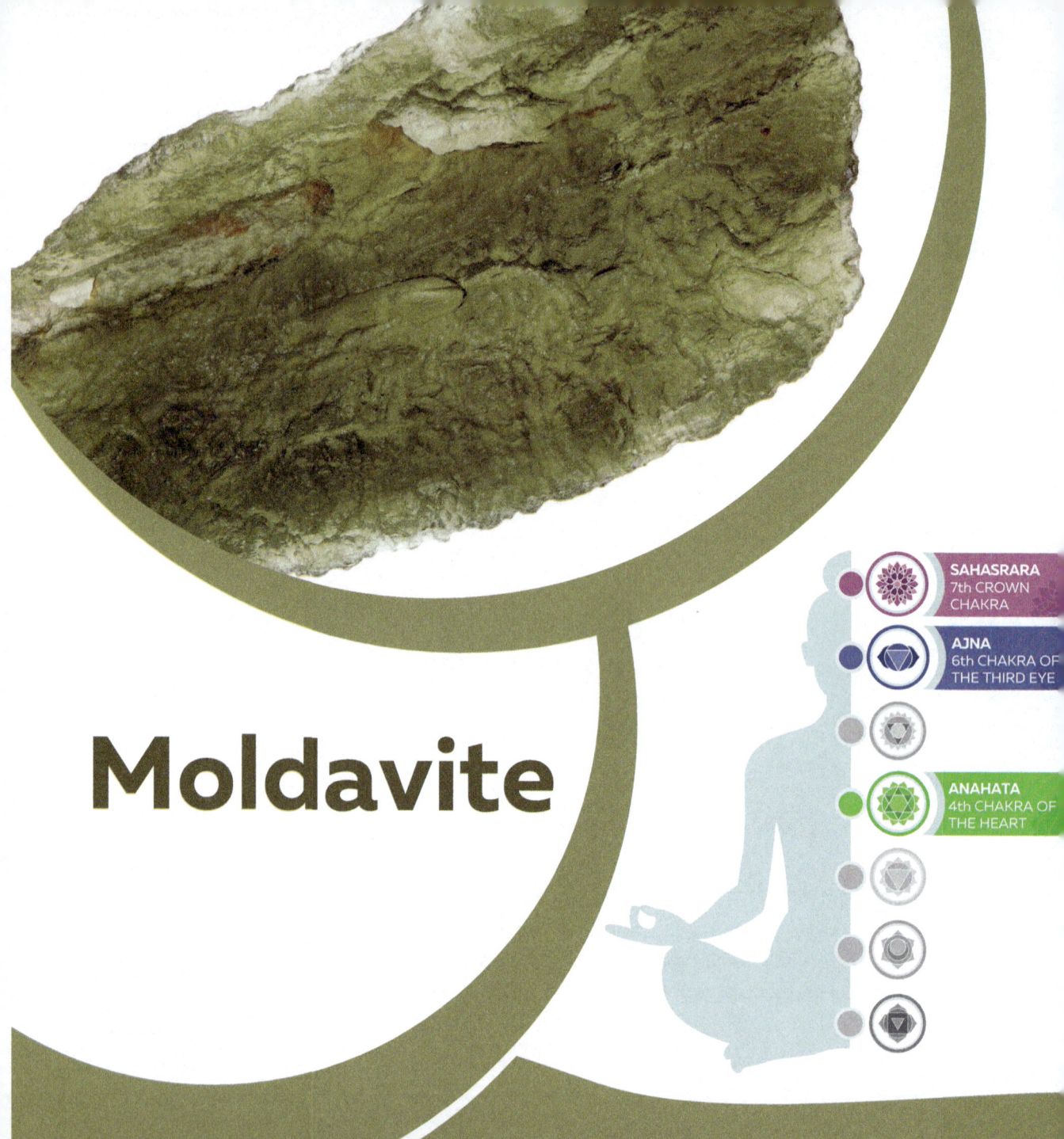

Colors:
Green

Crystal structure:
Amorphous

Zodiac sign:
All zodiac signs benefit from its properties, as it is a stone fallen from the stars.

History:
Moldavite is the result of the solidification of a meteorite that crashed into the Earth 15 million years ago. It was used as early as Egyptian times to get in touch with deities.

Properties:
Helps increase self-confidence, resolve emotional problems as well as combat anxiety and depression.

Body benefits:
Strengthens the immune system and gives strong support for the treatment of chronic diseases. Restores health and vitality; also helps with digestion-related problems and cardiovascular disease.

Mind and spirit benefits:
Strengthens connections with the universe, as well as increases creativity, memory, and concentration.

How to treat the stone:
To charge it, we can expose it to both sunlight and moonlight, and we can purify it with water.

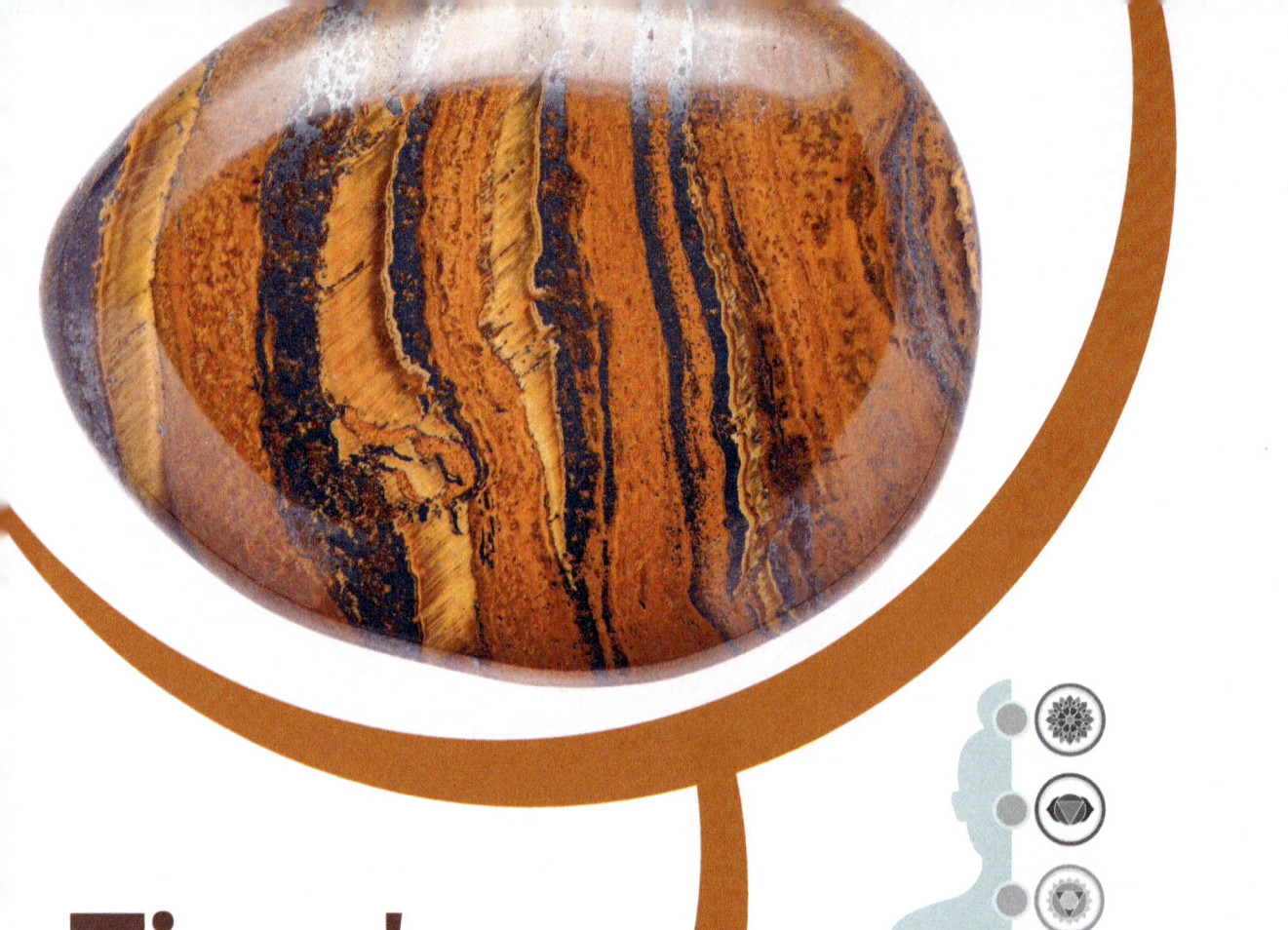

Tiger's eye

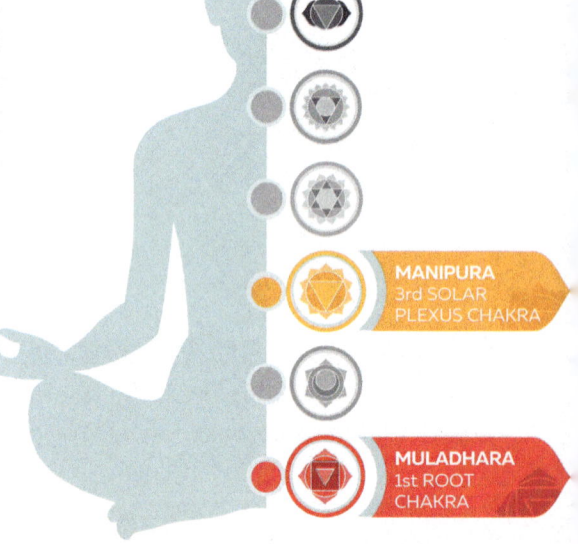

MANIPURA 3rd SOLAR PLEXUS CHAKRA

MULADHARA 1st ROOT CHAKRA

Colors:
Brown, Yellow-Gold, Black, Blue

Crystal structure:
Trigonal

Zodiac sign:
Gemini, Aries, Leo, Virgo

History:
The tiger's eye is a very famous stone among the stories of ancient peoples: for the Egyptians, it gave protection to the earth and the sun. According to Eastern mythology, it was linked to the animal considered the king, namely the tiger. Finally, the Romans used it to protect themselves from wounds.

Properties:
It is supportive in facing sudden change by giving us strength and courage. It also teaches us to move beyond pride and jealousy.

Body benefits:
Improves blood circulation, stimulates fertility, and balances the two hemispheres of the brain.

Mind and spirit benefits:
Attracts wealth and money in the key to personal growth, with the acquisition of skills that can be resold.

How to treat the stone:
To charge this stone, we can use an amethyst druse or expose it to moonlight overnight; we can then clean it with water.

Onyx

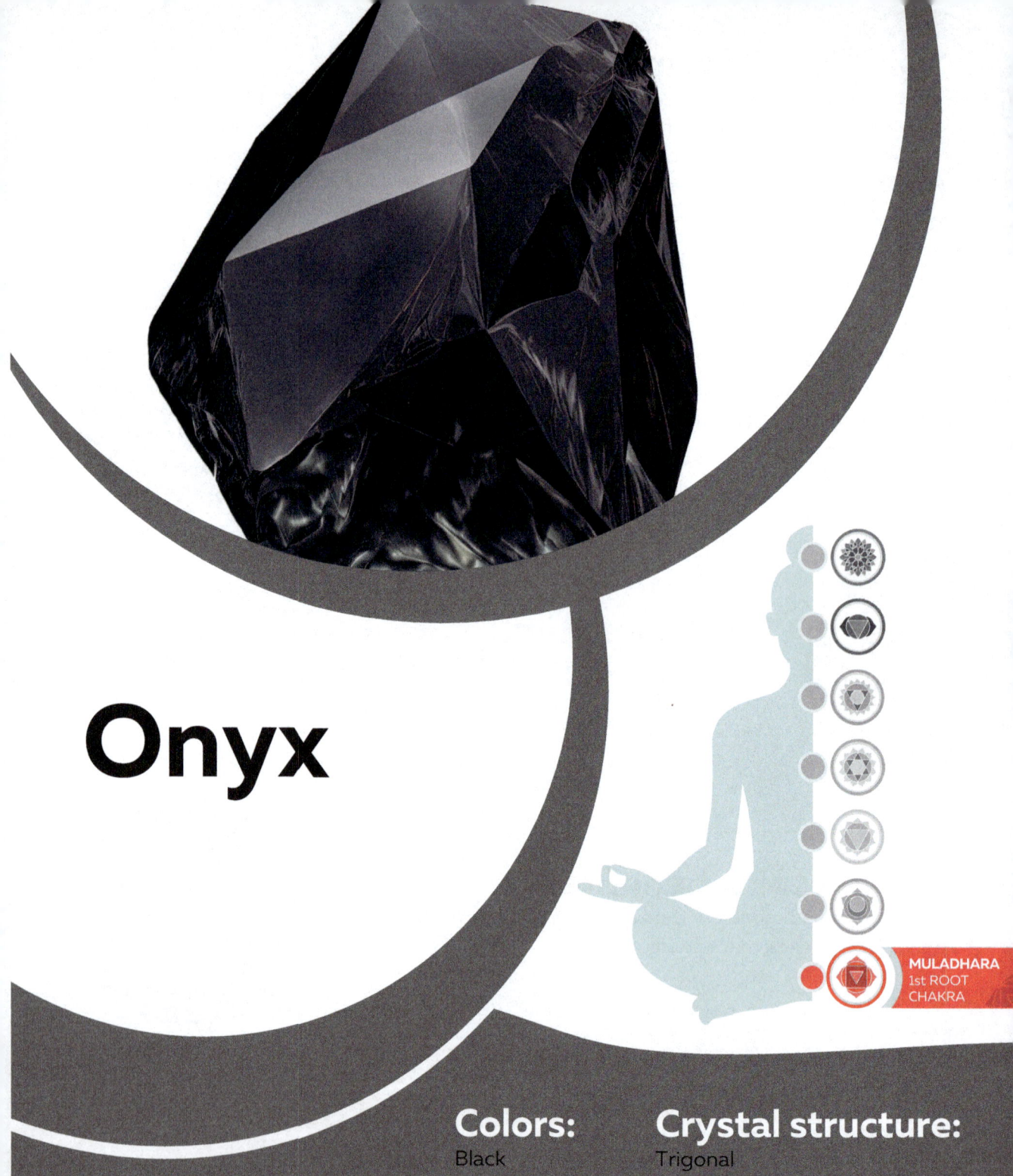

Colors:
Black

Crystal structure:
Trigonal

Zodiac sign:
Capricorn

MULADHARA
1st ROOT CHAKRA

History:
The meaning attributed to onyx is the Gem of Saturn, the planet of karma that reigns supreme over the law of cause-and-effect: so you get what you give.

Properties:
It highlights our strength and determination, making us feel invincible, showing ourselves differently to others and the world at large, and a guide that will help us achieve all our goals.

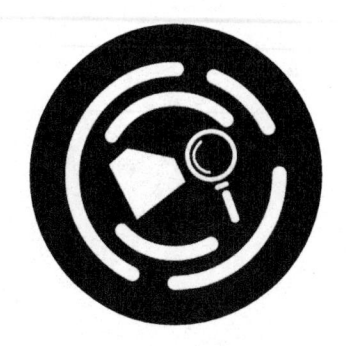

Body benefits:
Used to manage sexual impulses and to enhance sensuality and affection, promoting harmonious relationships and warding off temptations.

Mind and spirit benefits:
Helps to let go of feelings of grief and depression to welcome hope and positivity.

How to treat the stone:
We can use a soft cloth to cleanse the onyx in order to avoid discoloration and color buildup of the stone.

Fire opal

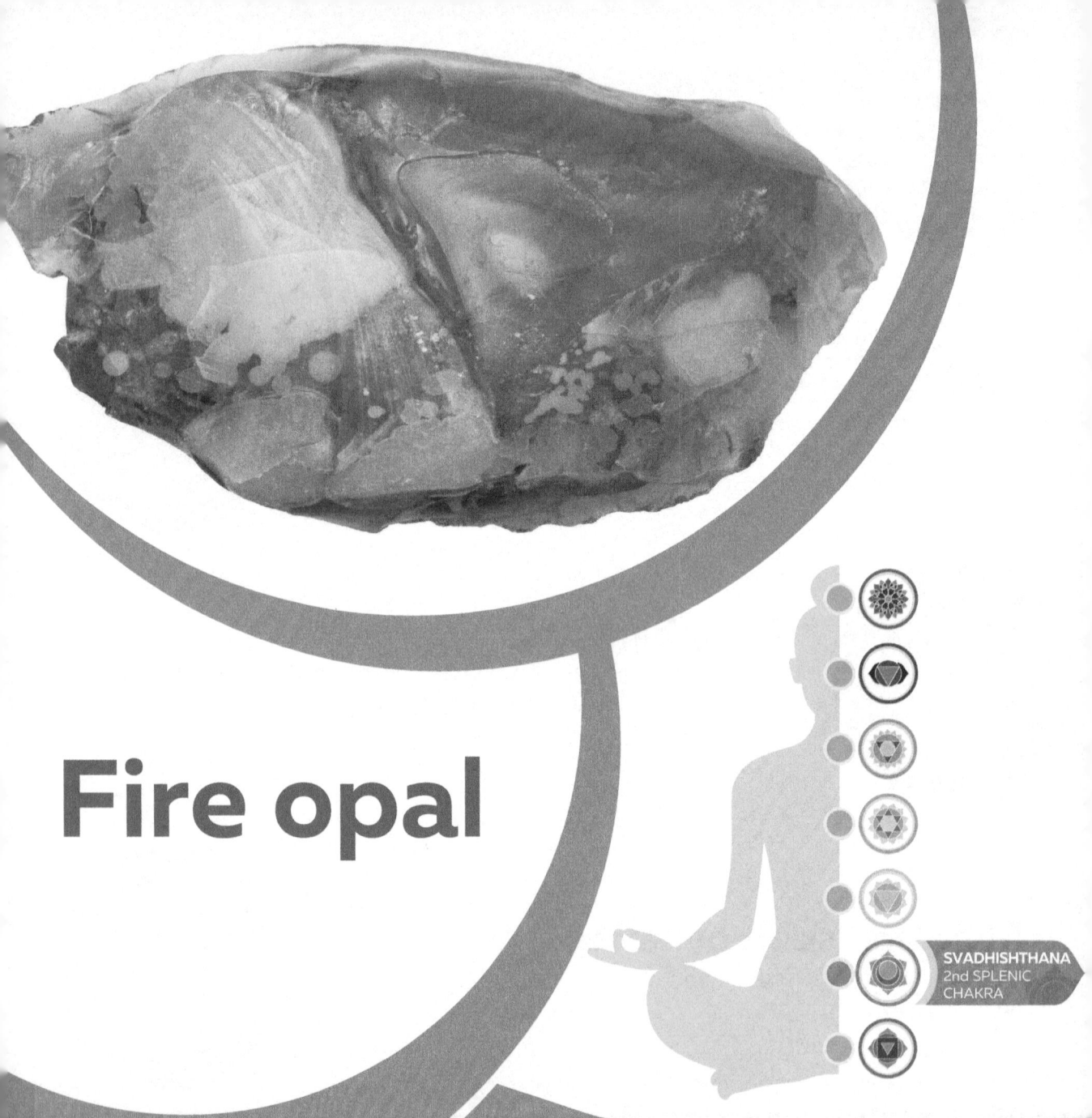

Colors:
Orange

Crystal structure:
Amorphous

Zodiac sign:
Libra, Scorpio

SVADHISHTHANA
2nd SPLENIC
CHAKRA

History:
It was discovered in Mexico and was used as early as Mayan and Aztec times; they collected this stone near volcanoes and made talismans from it to use in rituals as a catalyst for inner energy.

Properties:
Its purpose is to activate our mind by making us more dynamic and receptive, help us to have more courage, and activate our inner energy.

Body benefits:
It helps in the production of adrenaline and, just like other stones of this color, stimulates the sexual organs.

Mind and spirit benefits:
It helps us find the courage within ourselves to overcome difficult situations or new challenges.

How to treat the stone:
To purify fire opal, we can use incense, a block of clay, earth, and a quartz druse, while to charge it, we can use other crystals such as rock crystal, hyaline quartz, or citrine quartz.

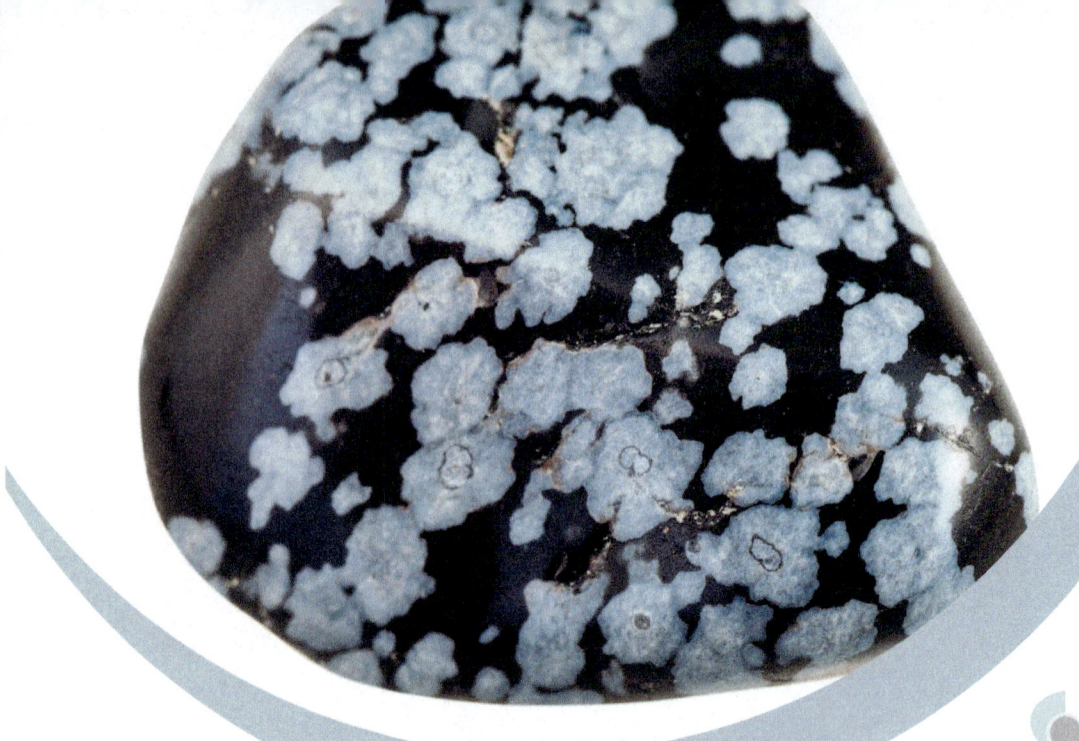

Obsidian snowflake

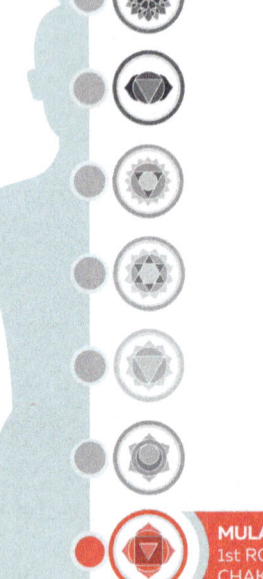

Colors:
Black with white bows

Crystal structure:
Amorphous

Zodiac sign:
Capricorn, Sagittarius

MULADHARA
1st ROOT CHAKRA

80

History:
According to the oldest legends, snowflake obsidian has the power to cast out demons, which is why it was used by Mayan priests during magic rituals.

Properties:
Works on feminine energy and connects it to the earth, giving us balance and leading us to work with our inner self in an introspective sense.

Body benefits:
Perfect to use as a protective amulet because it helps fight fears of all kinds.

Mind and spirit benefits:
Provides support when we fail to make progress, stimulates the desire for adventure, and instills confidence in facing challenges.

How to treat the stone:
To charge this stone we can leave it overnight under the influences of the Moon or use running water or, again, smoke from a holy pole.

Moonstone

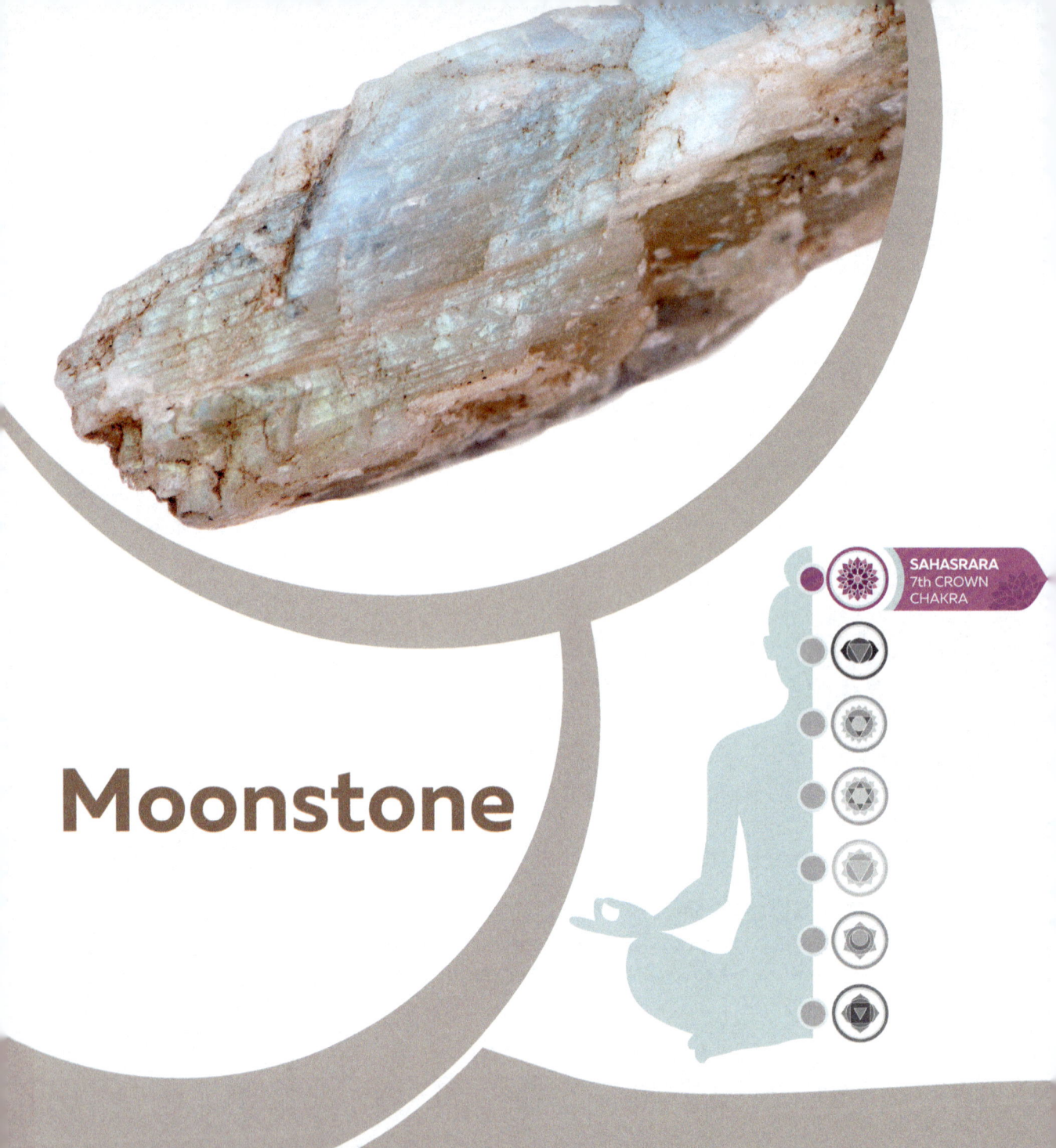

SAHASRARA 7th CROWN CHAKRA

Colors:
White

Crystal structure:
Monoclinic

Zodiac sign:
Cancer, Virgo, Gemini

History:
Moonstone has always been associated with the Moon and femininity. It has been used for centuries and was attributed various properties and virtues, especially that of saving from storms at sea and being a good luck charm for those sailing.

Properties:
This stone has the power to align you with spiritual energies and allows you to get in touch with your unconscious.

Body benefits:
Due to the feminine energy, it has a beneficial effect on the female genital system, soothes menstrual pain, and is also recommended for menopause.

Mind and spirit benefits:
Promotes optimism and enables us to deal with changes in the right way. Good luck to those who love to travel, especially sea travelers.

How to treat the stone:
To purify it, we can use real incense, or we can leave it submerged in water so that it is also charged.

Citrine Quartz

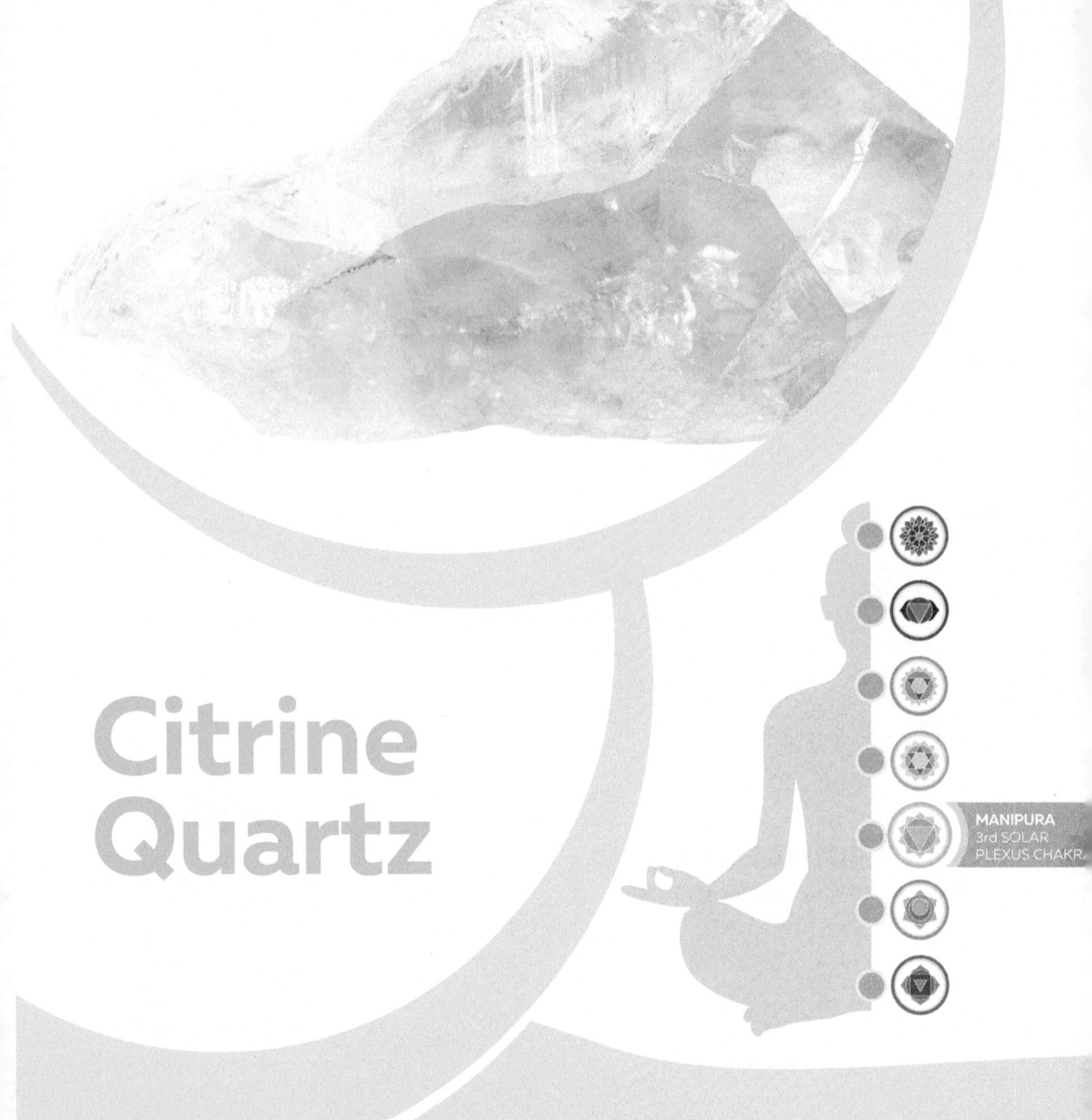

MANIPURA
3rd SOLAR
PLEXUS CHAKR.

Colors:
Yellow

Crystal structure:
Trigonal

Zodiac sign:
Gemini, Leo, Libra, Virgo

84

History:
It has always been considered the stone of health. It was used to cure snake venoms. In the Middle East, this stone was believed to promote good fortune and maintain wealth, so merchants used to keep stones along with money.

Properties:
It is the stone of the sun and attracts all positive, beneficial, active things around us.

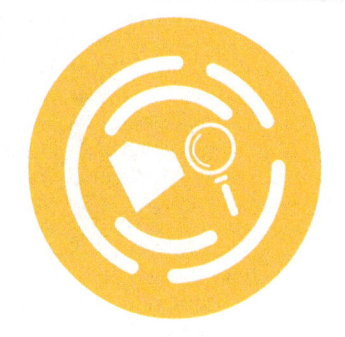

Body benefits:
Suitable for athletes because it gives energy, keeps performance high, fights fatigue, and promotes digestion.

Mind and spirit benefits:
It gives vitality and energy and is an incentive to turn our projects into concrete ideas. Placed in the center of a room, it energizes the whole room.

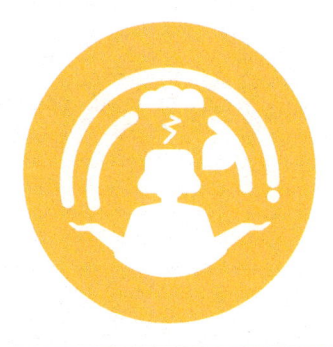

How to treat the stone:
No need to purify it as it does not attract negative energies. You can leave it in running water for a few minutes.

Smoked quartz

MULADHARA
1st ROOT CHAKRA

Colors:
Brown, Black, Dark gray

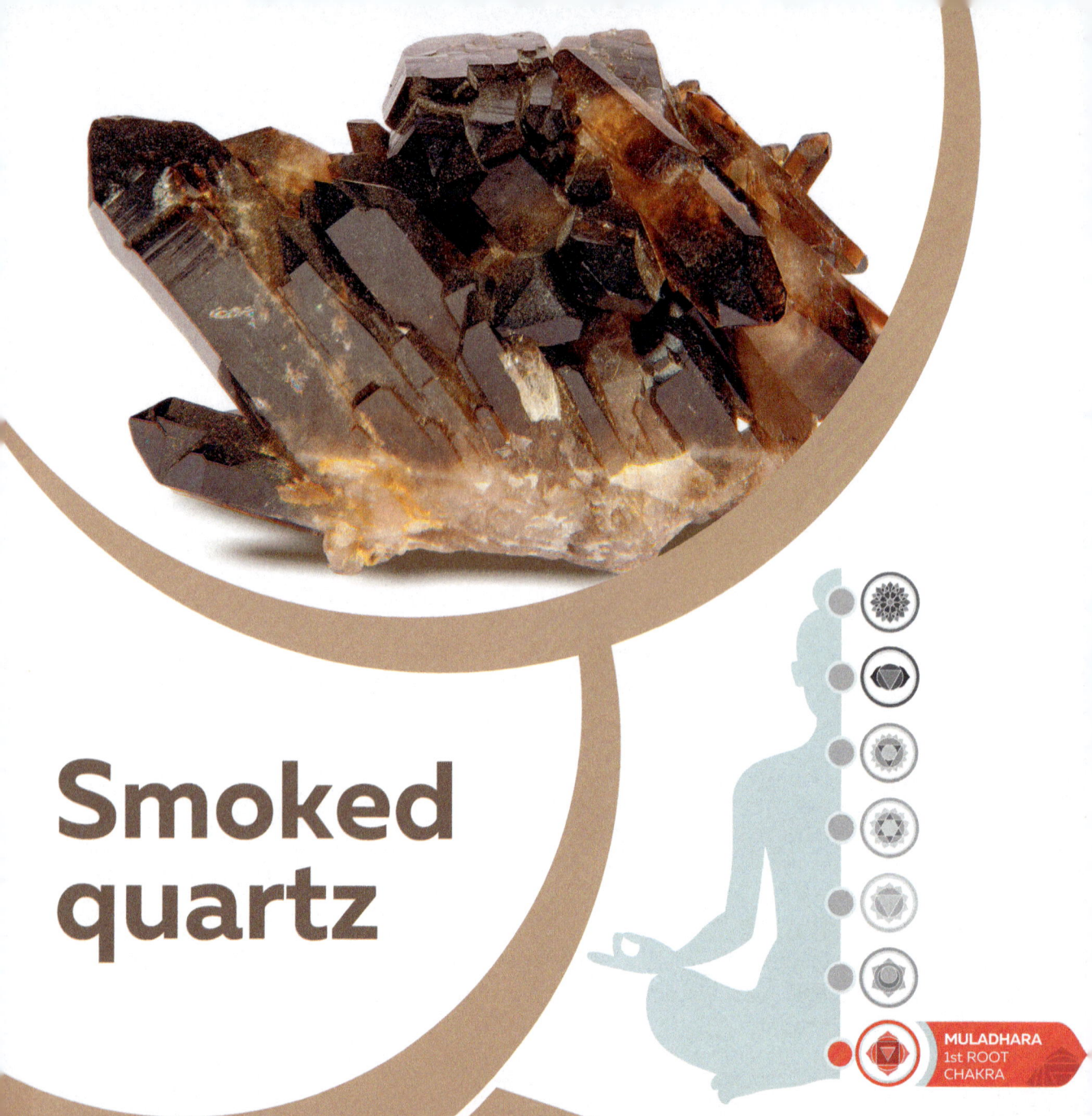

Crystal structure:
Trigonal

Zodiac sign:
Taurus, Scorpio, Libra

History:
Legends have it that smoky quartz holds within it the power of earthbound deities: even the Romans used it to overcome the pain they experienced in unpleasant situations such as mourning. In shamanic rituals, it is used to connect with the spirits of the underworld.

Properties:
It helps us ward off fears and stress, combat panic attacks and anxiety, and shape the reality we live in to fit our aspirations.

Body benefits:
Relieves chronic pain, especially that related to the upper body, and fights radiation.

Mind and spirit benefits:
Used to protect us against the negativity of the environments in which we live and restores calm in stressful situations.

How to treat the stone:
To purify it, we can use natural incense or an amethyst druse, while to charge it, we can expose it to direct moonlight or non-direct sunlight.

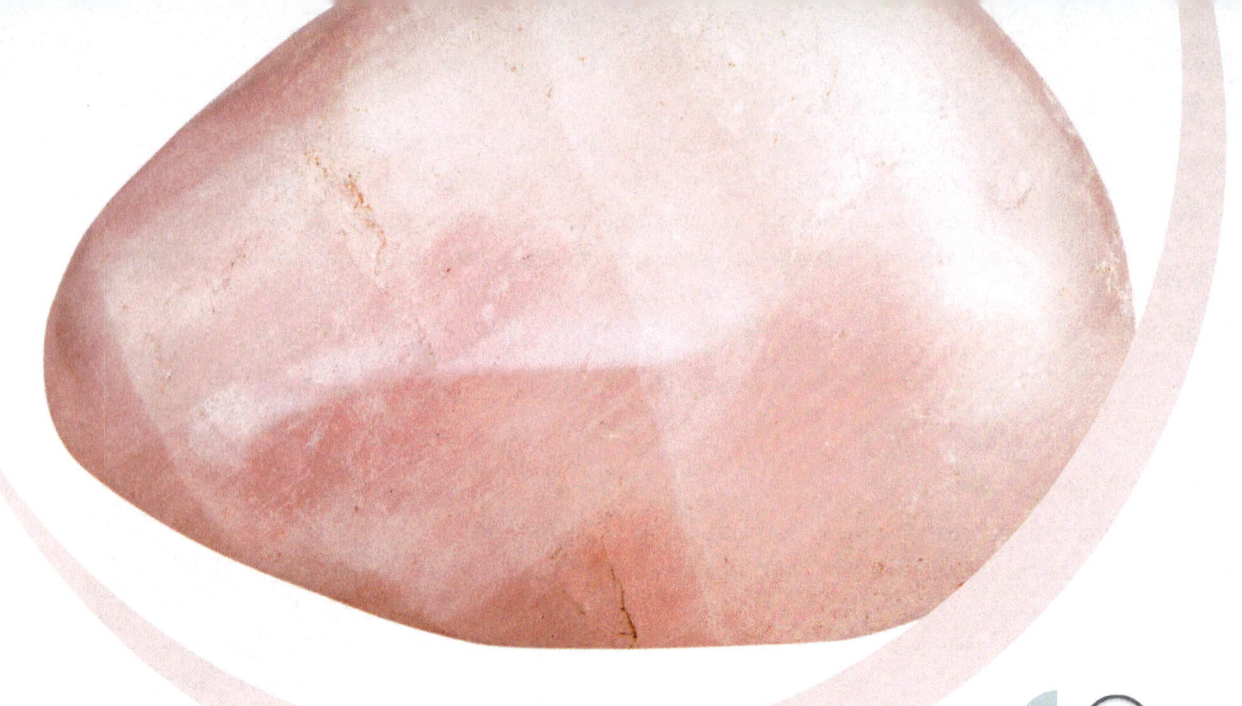

Rose quartz

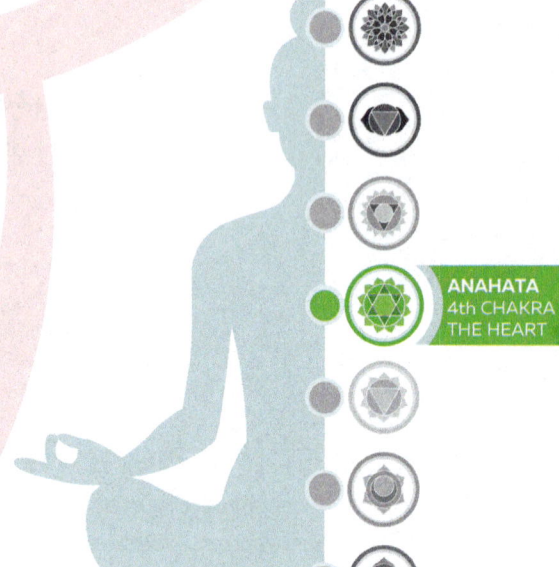

ANAHATA
4th CHAKRA OF THE HEART

Colors:
Pink

Crystal structure:
Trigonal

Zodiac sign:
Virgo, Cancer, Libra

History:
Legends related to rose quartz are obviously related to Aphrodite and Gaia as a symbol of love and fertility.

Properties:
It helps to recognize our most hidden talents and get us back on track whenever we no longer know who we are.

Body benefits:
Wearing it as a necklace at the level of the heart, this mineral helps to eliminate negative emotions and energies that have settled in our hearts over time; it helps to love without fear.

Mind and spirit benefits:
It relieves wounds caused by lack of love and mitigates feelings of loneliness. It is also able to dissolve heavy energies from underground, perhaps from waterways or geological faults that affect the rhythm of the body's cells.

How to treat the stone:
We can purify rose quartz with real incense or by simply laying it on an amethyst druse, and we can charge it with running water.

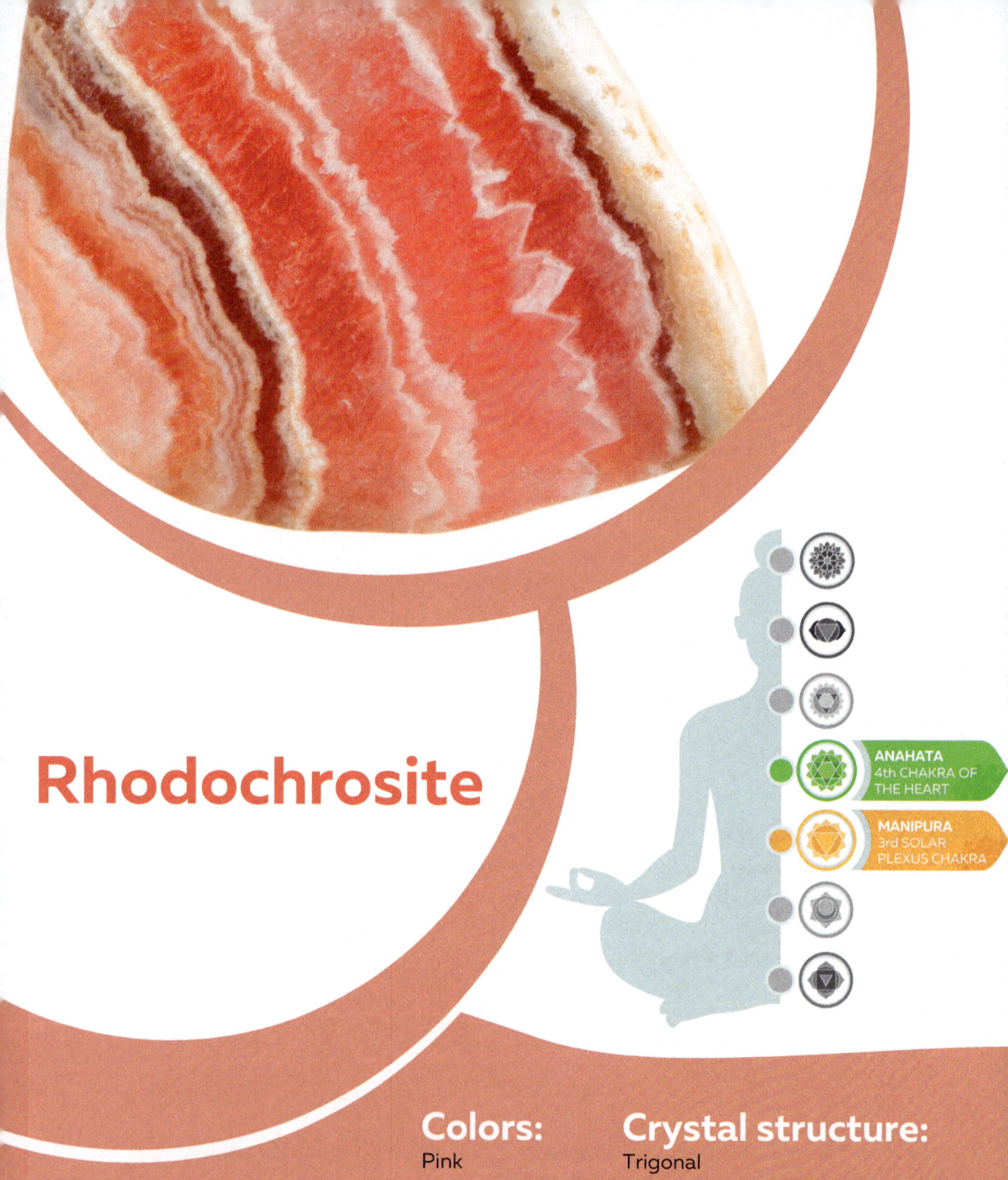

Rhodochrosite

Colors:
Pink

Crystal structure:
Trigonal

Zodiac sign:
Cancer, Scorpio, Libra

ANAHATA
4th CHAKRA OF THE HEART

MANIPURA
3rd SOLAR PLEXUS CHAKRA

History:
Rhodochrosite comes from the Greek rhodon, meaning "rose," and from chrosis, meaning "colored." According to legend, the Incas believed that this stone was the blood of ancestors turned to stone.

Properties:
The strength this stone can impart to us is unparalleled, as we will find ourselves picking up the pieces and getting back on our feet with almost no effort. It is used to give us security and integrity.

Body benefits:
It will awaken the child in us, inspiring a joyful and playful attitude toward life, attracting compassion, and repairing emotional rifts we may have developed in the course of relationships.

Mind and spirit benefits:
It is able to shine the light of love, make us examine old wounds, and make us compassionate toward ourselves.

How to treat the stone:
To recharge it, we can use an amethyst druse, or moonlight, to avoid sunlight.

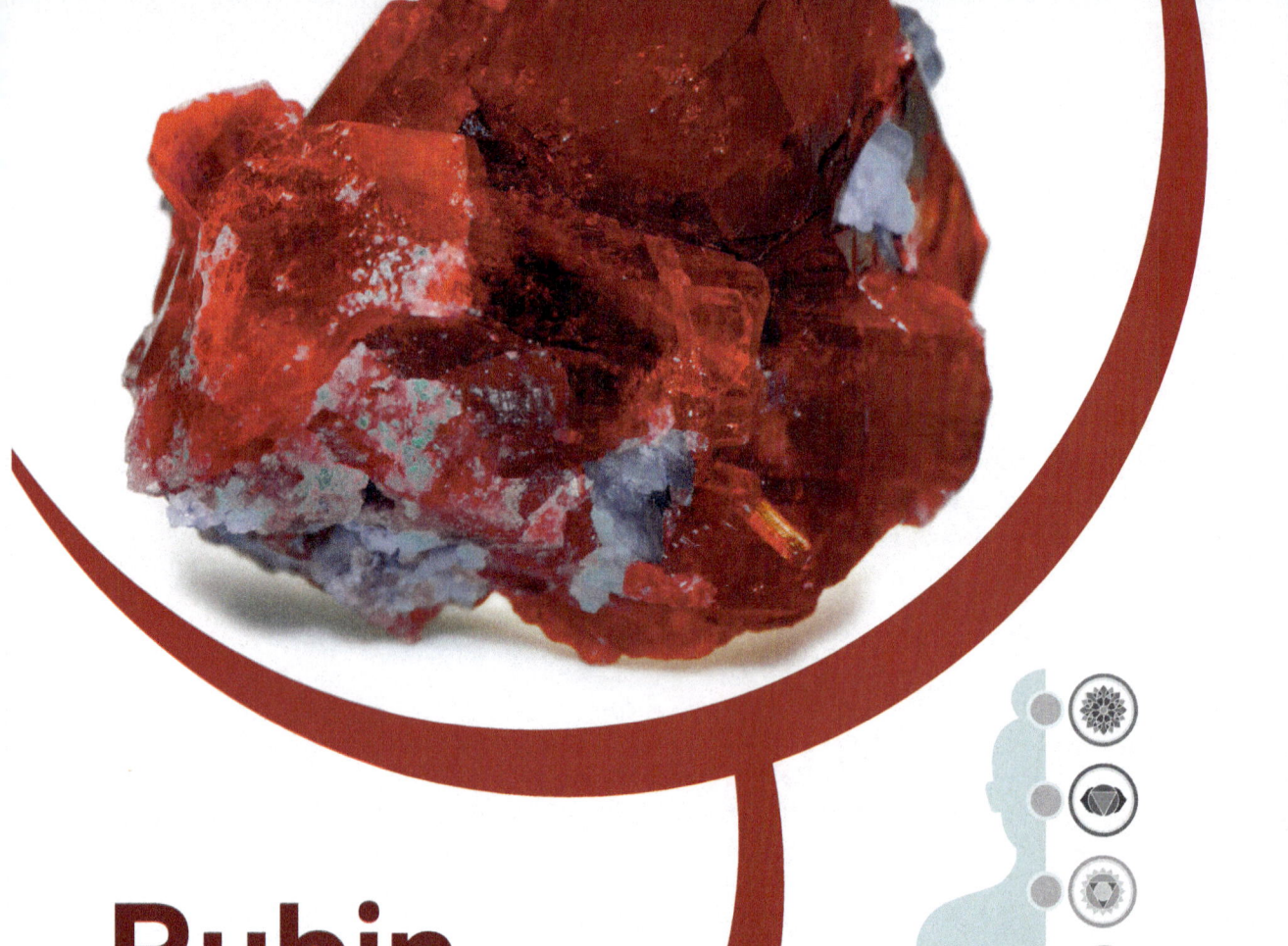

Rubin

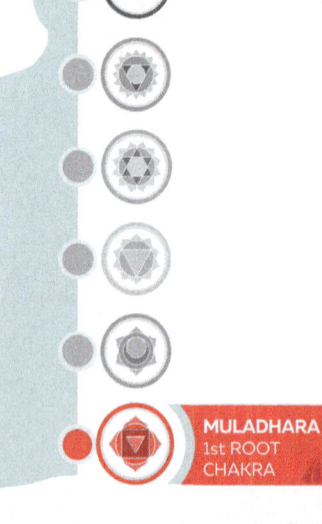

Colors:
Red

Crystal structure:
Trigonal

Zodiac sign:
Aries, Leo, Scorpio

MULADHARA
1st ROOT CHAKRA

History:
It has always been considered the stone of passion and, according to various legends, was believed to burn an unquenchable flame inside.

Properties:
Ruby promotes sexual desire and energy, improves partner attunement and enhances the ability to conceive.

Body benefits:
It is used to treat fertility problems and impotence. It promotes the circulation of lymph and blood.

Mind and spirit benefits:
Promotes concentration and determination. Brings warmth and energy to environments.

How to treat the stone:
To purify it, use incense or an amethyst druse. To charge it, avoid sunlight and moonlight; the other methods are all suitable.

Selenite

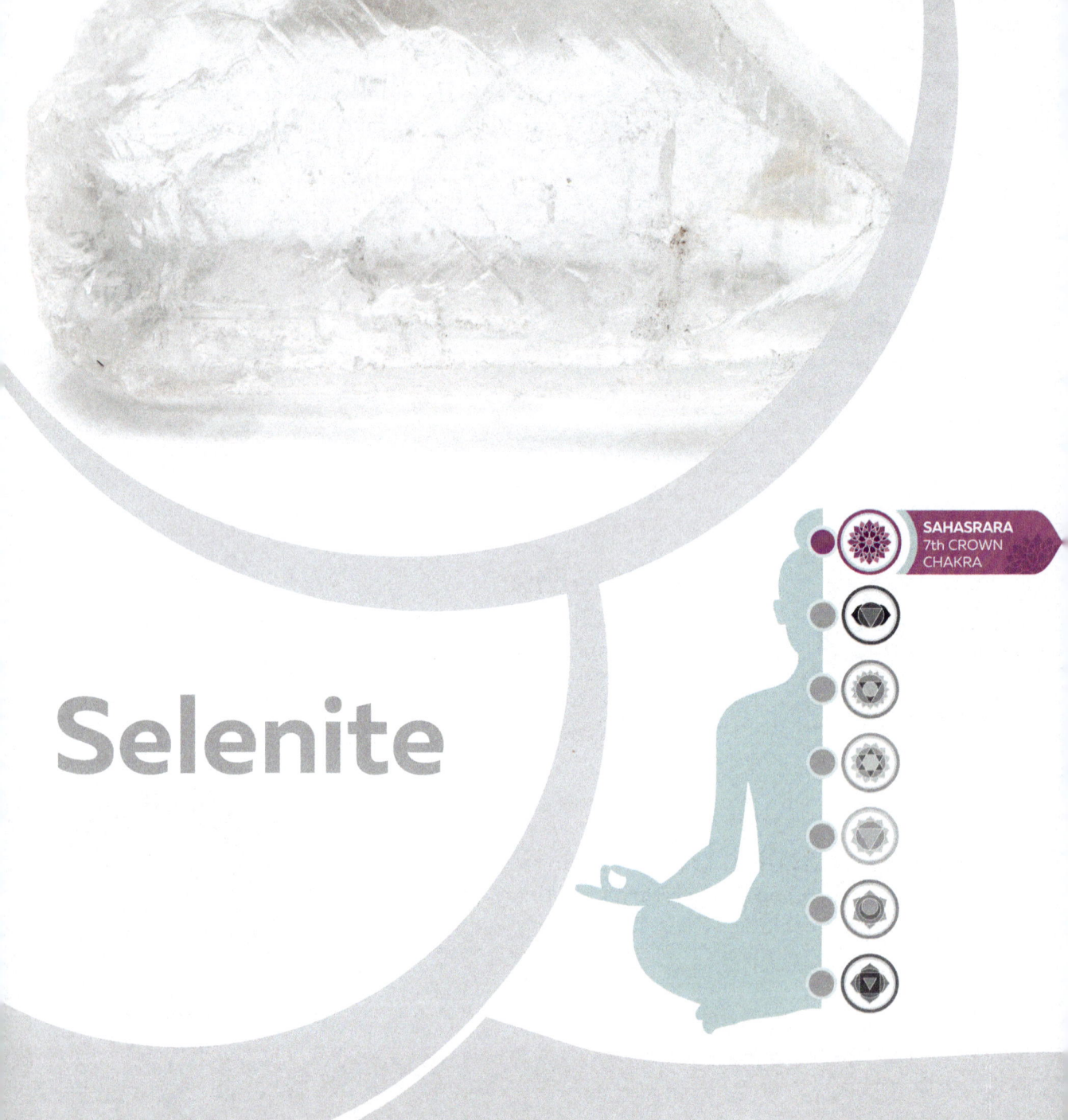

SAHASRARA 7th CROWN CHAKRA

Colors:
White

Crystal structure:
Monoclinic

Zodiac sign:
Cancer, Aquarius

History:
The legends related to selenite involve the earliest peoples placing the stone in places where there was a sick person or creating a compound used to mark on doors the place where the sick rested.

Properties:
It is related to feelings, women, and is used as a support during times of change; it has a great ability to put us in touch with divine protectors and spirit guides.

Body benefits:
It helps us act on confusing emotional states, as it dampens our strength, giving us great stability that counteracts mood swings.

Mind and spirit benefits:
It is used to eliminate negative energies and encourages introspective reflection on life and events we have already experienced, causing us to grow spiritually. It is perfect for those who are always guided by rigid patterns.

How to treat the stone:
To purify it, we can use fumigation with incense, while to charge it, we can expose it to moonlight.

Emerald

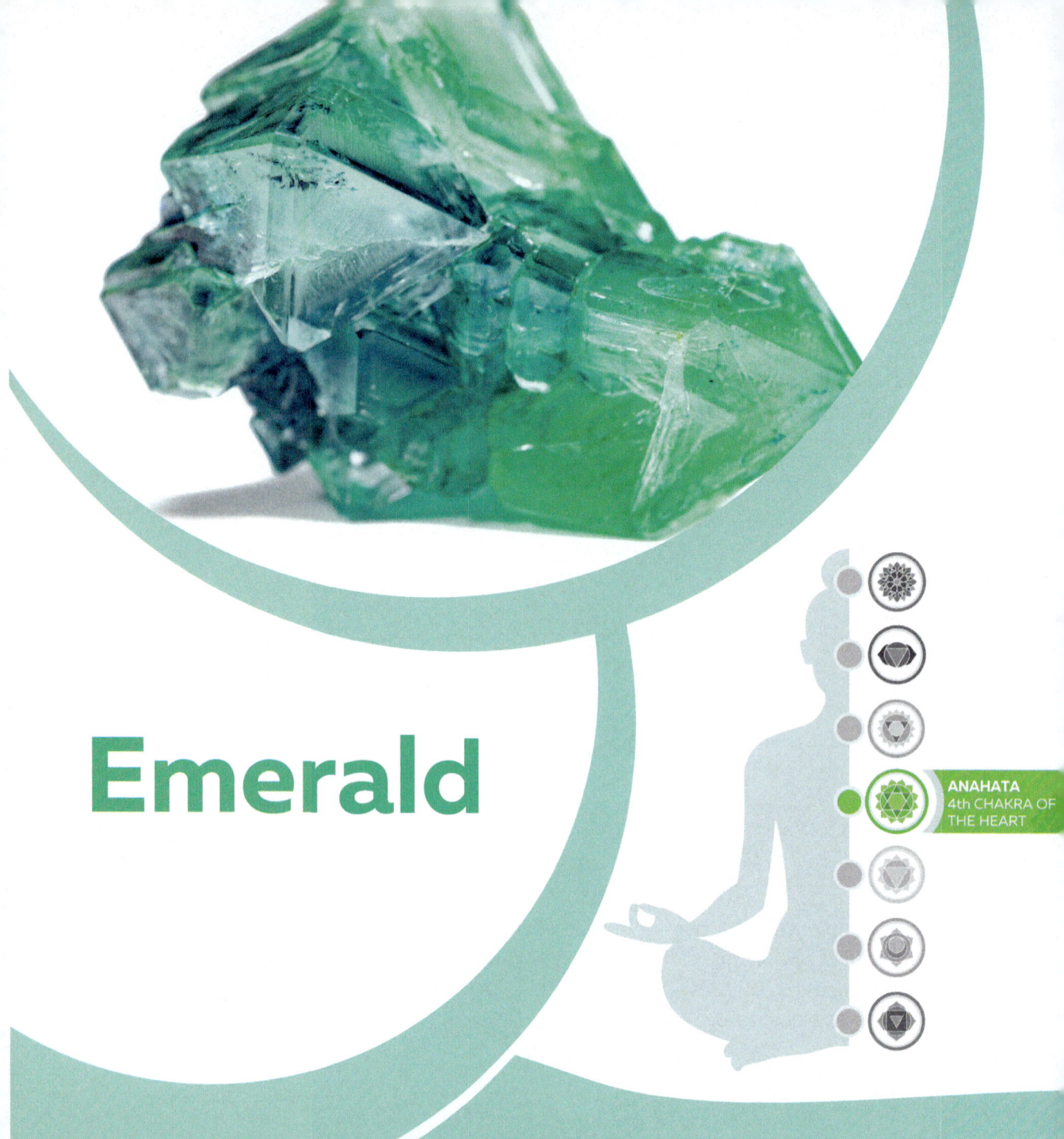

ANAHATA
4th CHAKRA OF THE HEART

Colors:
Green

Crystal structure:
Hexagonal

Zodiac sign:
Cancer, Libra, Capricorn

History:
In ancient times, it was believed that emeralds, precisely because of their purity, were able to sense betrayal, which is why it was customary to give them to brides. Such a pure jewel would not tolerate "impure" gestures and would shatter, thus revealing betrayal.

Properties:
Its benefits are still appreciated for curing diseases because its vibrations absolve purification and balance. Thanks to this crystal, we can attract loyalty, happiness, and balance between partners.

Body benefits:
Heals disorders of the respiratory system, liver, and lungs and has a beneficial effect on the eyes. It protects the heart and detoxifies the liver and kidneys.

Mind and spirit benefits:
It provides us with great strength to deal with life's problems and our emotions, strengthens our memory, and facilitates divination.

How to treat the stone:
Purify it with salt or earth. To charge it instead, simply expose it to moonlight.

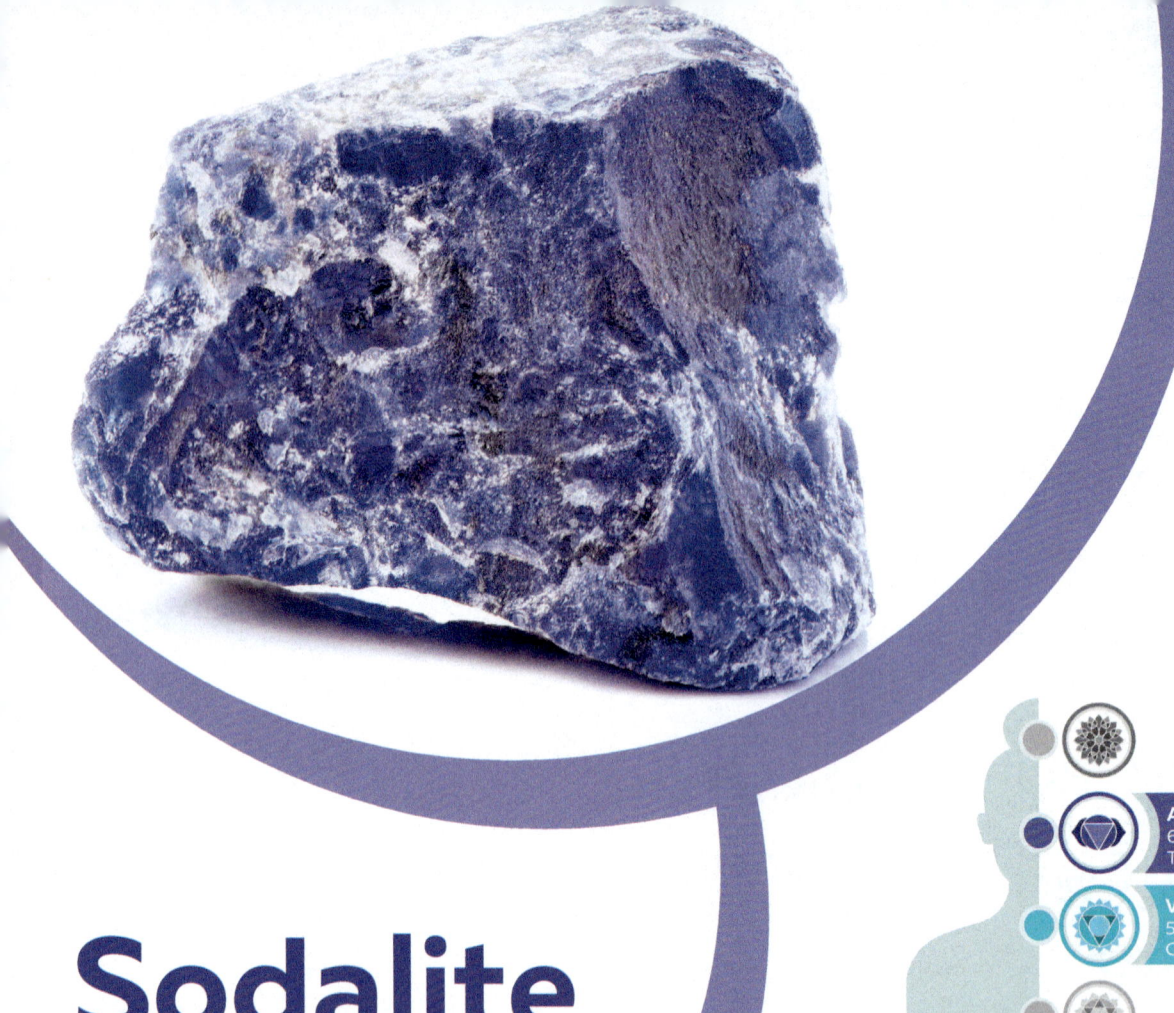

Sodalite

AJNA
6th CHAKRA OF THE THIRD EYE

VISHUDDHA
5th THROAT CHAKRA

Colors:
Blue

Crystal structure:
Cubic

Zodiac sign:
Gemini, Sagittarius

History:
According to a legend told in South America, a woman who was in love with a man who did not love her took her own life, and when the man found out what he had caused, he wept in despair; from the fusion of his tears with the deep blue color of the sky, sodalite was born.

Properties:
It is the stone of logic and rationality and calms the mind to help ward off fears and guilt. It helps to communicate calmly and get clarity about one's thoughts.

Body benefits:
Strengthens the immune system and protects against common diseases, speeds up metabolism, and improves digestion.

Mind and spirit benefits:
Helps organize thought and brings clarity to the inner self. Placed in the room, it promotes meditation and aids in relaxation.

How to treat the stone:
Purify it with incense, clay, or an amethyst druse. To charge it, expose it to the Moon's rays.

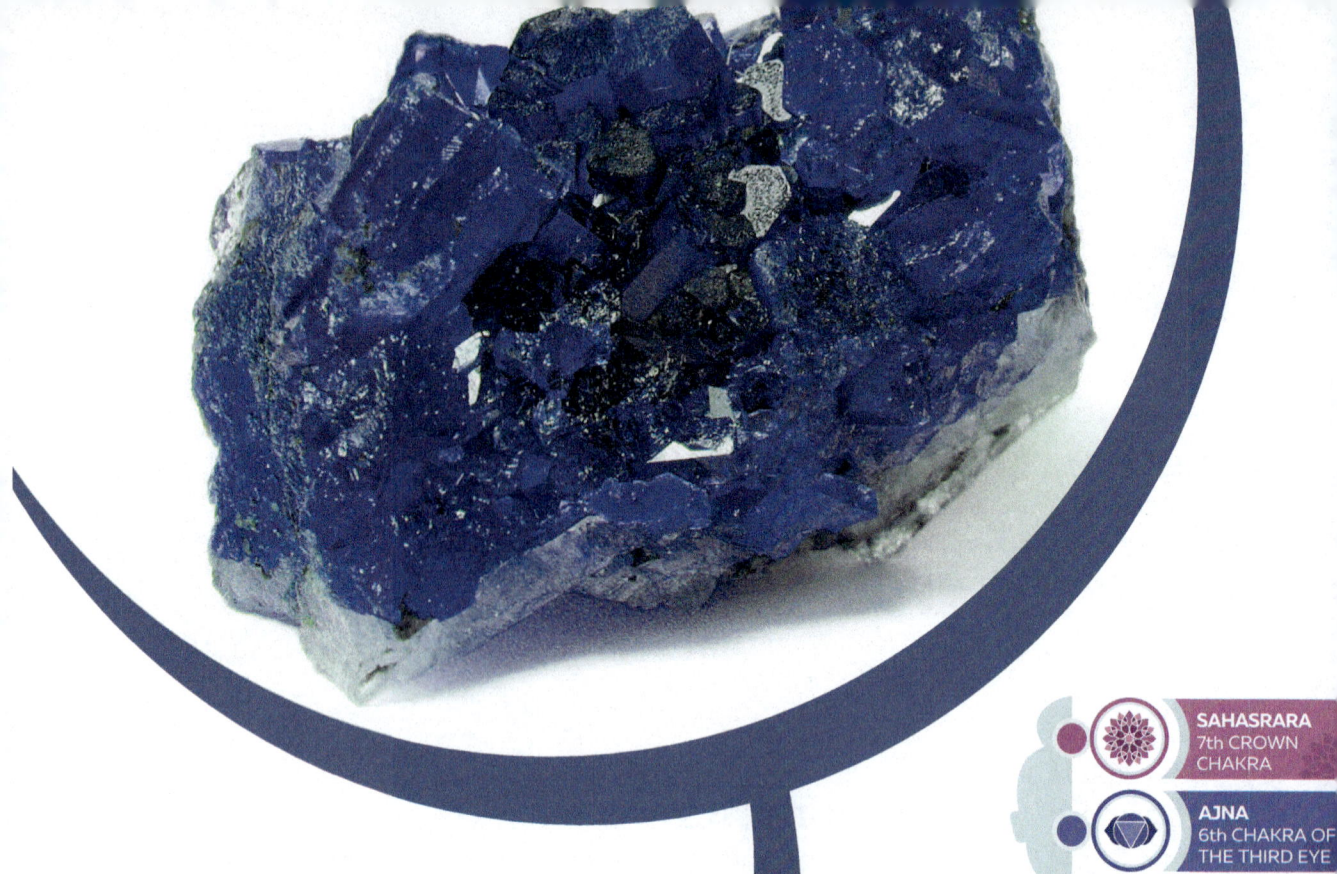

Tanzanite

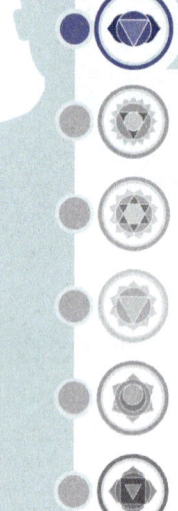

SAHASRARA
7th CROWN CHAKRA

AJNA
6th CHAKRA OF THE THIRD EYE

Colors:
Blue with Purple highlights

Crystal structure:
Rhombic

Zodiac sign:
Sagittarius

100

History:
It was discovered in the 1960s in Tanzania by a pastor, hence its name. It is a very rare stone, found only in a deposit at the foot of Kilimanjaro, which is why it is much rarer than a diamond.

Properties:
It is the symbol of the life cycle, evoking energy and helping to reach the spiritual side. Its energy acts as a link between the heart and the mind.

Body benefits:
Useful in treating the thyroid, strengthens the nervous system as well as promotes the work of the kidneys.

Mind and spirit benefits:
Helps bring calm to an overactive mind. Generates energy and happiness, and helps cope with emotional problems. Within the home, it helps strengthen family bonding.

How to treat the stone:
Purify with running water and charge with moonbeams.

101

Topaz

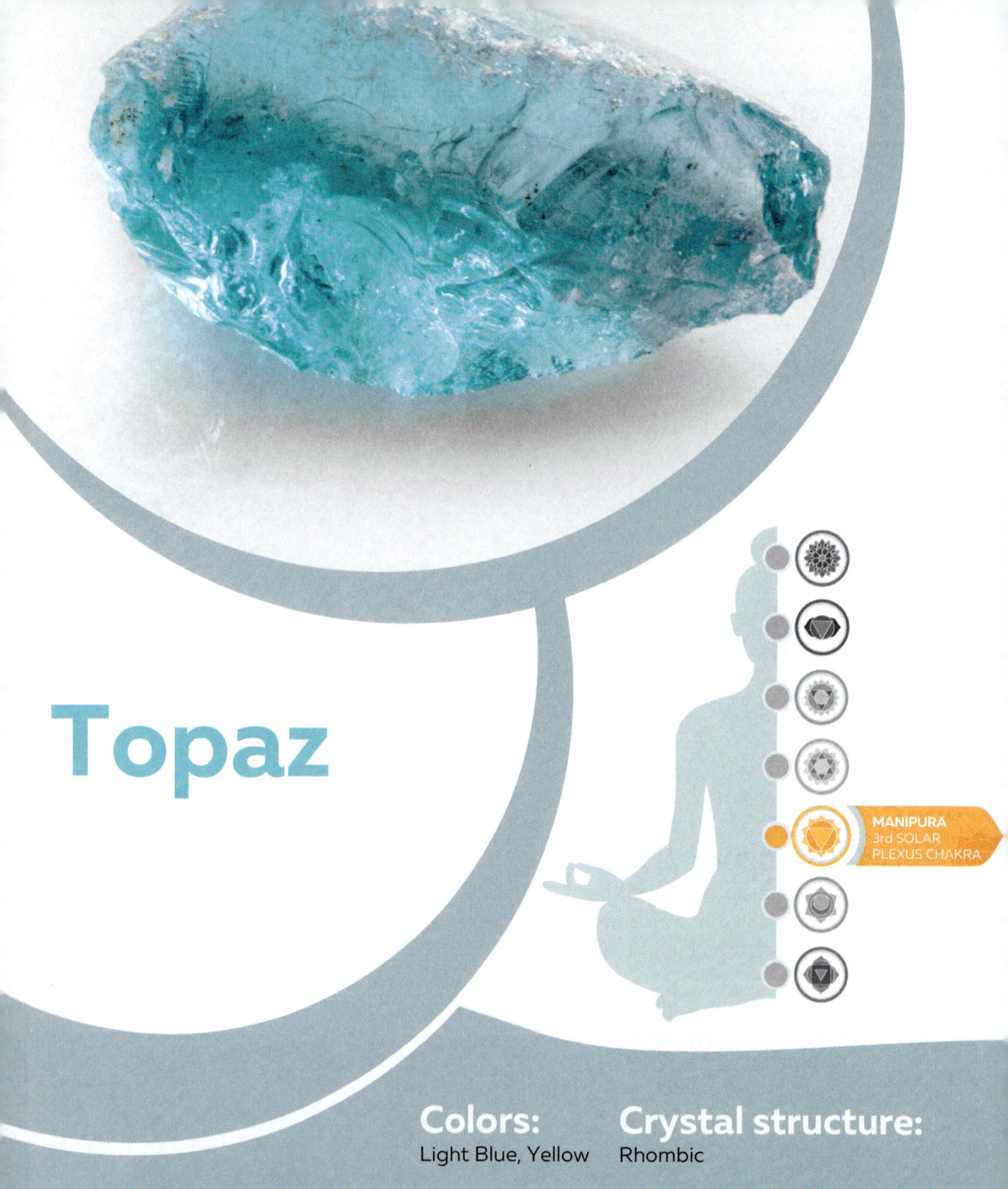

MANIPURA
3rd SOLAR
PLEXUS CHAKRA

Colors:
Light Blue, Yellow

Crystal structure:
Rhombic

Zodiac sign:
Taurus, Cancer, Leo, Virgo

102

History:
For Hindus, topaz was a sacred stone belonging to the Kepa Tree, and they believed that wearing this stone would extend life as well as sharpen the intellect.

Properties:
It is used to channel energies to help us keep a clearer mind as it works deeply on the mental sphere.

Body benefits:
Attracts wealth and helps us save money. Helps speed up metabolism.

Mind and spirit benefits:
Most useful when we need to undertake an inner quest and reinforces the practices, we are most excited about, such as meditation or yoga, as it brings greater awareness into our lives.

How to treat the stone:
To purify topaz, we can use an amethyst druse, or we can place it under the rays of the crescent Moon.

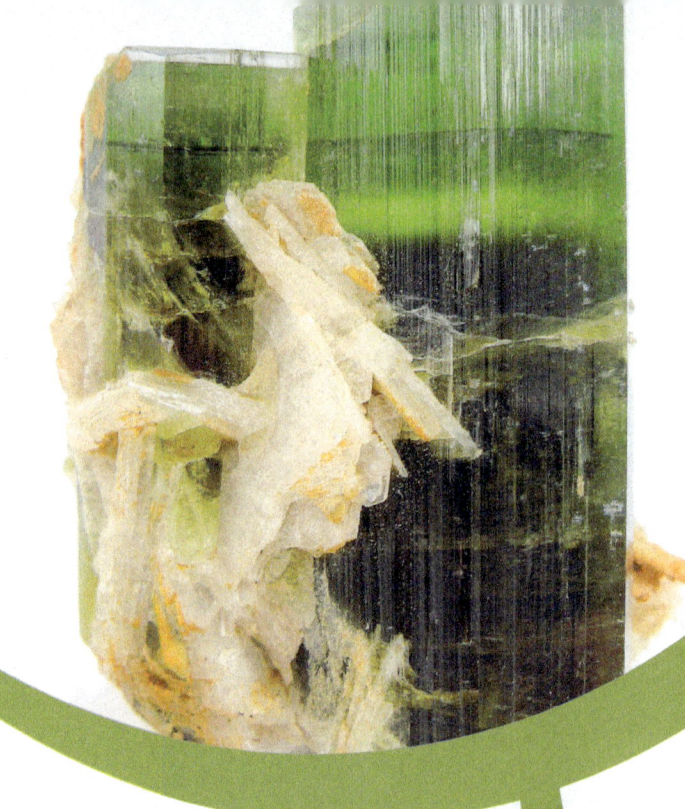

Green tourmaline

ANAHATA
4th CHAKRA OF THE HEART

Colors:
Green

Crystal structure:
Trigonal

Zodiac sign:
Cancer, Sagittarius

104

History:
Tourmaline is derived from tuḷadhi, meaning dark stone. In ancient times, green tourmaline was used to attract prosperity and protect against disease. It was also once used to overcome emotional blocks and improve relationships.

Properties:
This stone helps decrease anxiety and stress, bringing calm and peace back into our lives. It also helps improve concentration and mental clarity and enables us to overcome the fear of loneliness and abandonment.

Body benefits:
Reduces exhaustion and chronic fatigue. Strengthens the immune and nervous systems in addition to stimulating cell regeneration.

Mind and spirit benefits:
It helps us balance our emotions by overcoming emotional blocks and strengthening our self-confidence, as well as our ability to feel loved and appreciated.

How to treat the stone:
To purify it, we can use real incense or place it on a crystal geode.

Turquoise

VISHUDDHA
5th THROAT CHAKRA

Colors:
Green, Light Blue

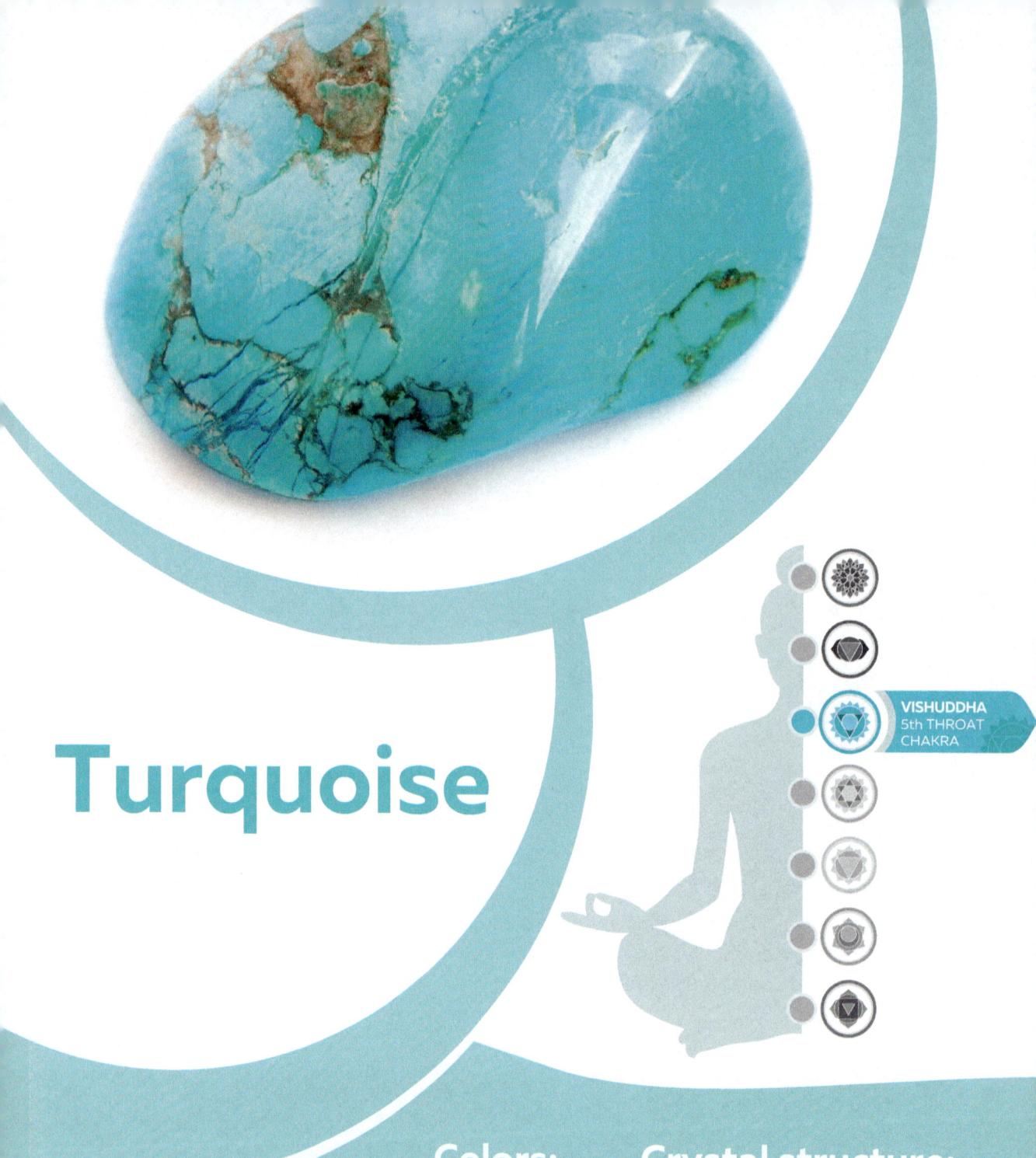

Crystal structure:
Triclinic

Zodiac sign:
Sagittarius, Aquarius

History:
Usually, this stone is given to the person one loves because it brings happiness and wealth. According to one legend, the color of the stone fades when the love for the person it is given to fades.

Properties:
It symbolizes wisdom and calmness, protects us from negativity, and offers us clearer thinking. It is considered the ultimate traveler's stone, as it protects against theft, falls, and accidents of various kinds.

Body benefits:
Solves problems related to vision and emotional imbalances. Suitable for those working at computers as it promotes mental relaxation.

Mind and spirit benefits:
Helps not to dwell on past mistakes or missed opportunities, control anger and avoid extremes.

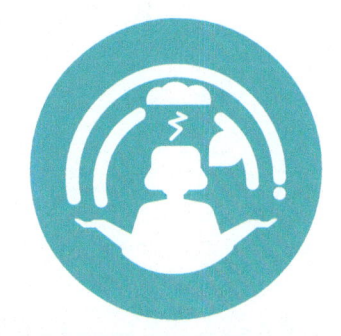

How to treat the stone:
This is a porous stone, capable of absorbing any liquid that comes in contact with it, so water would be best avoided.

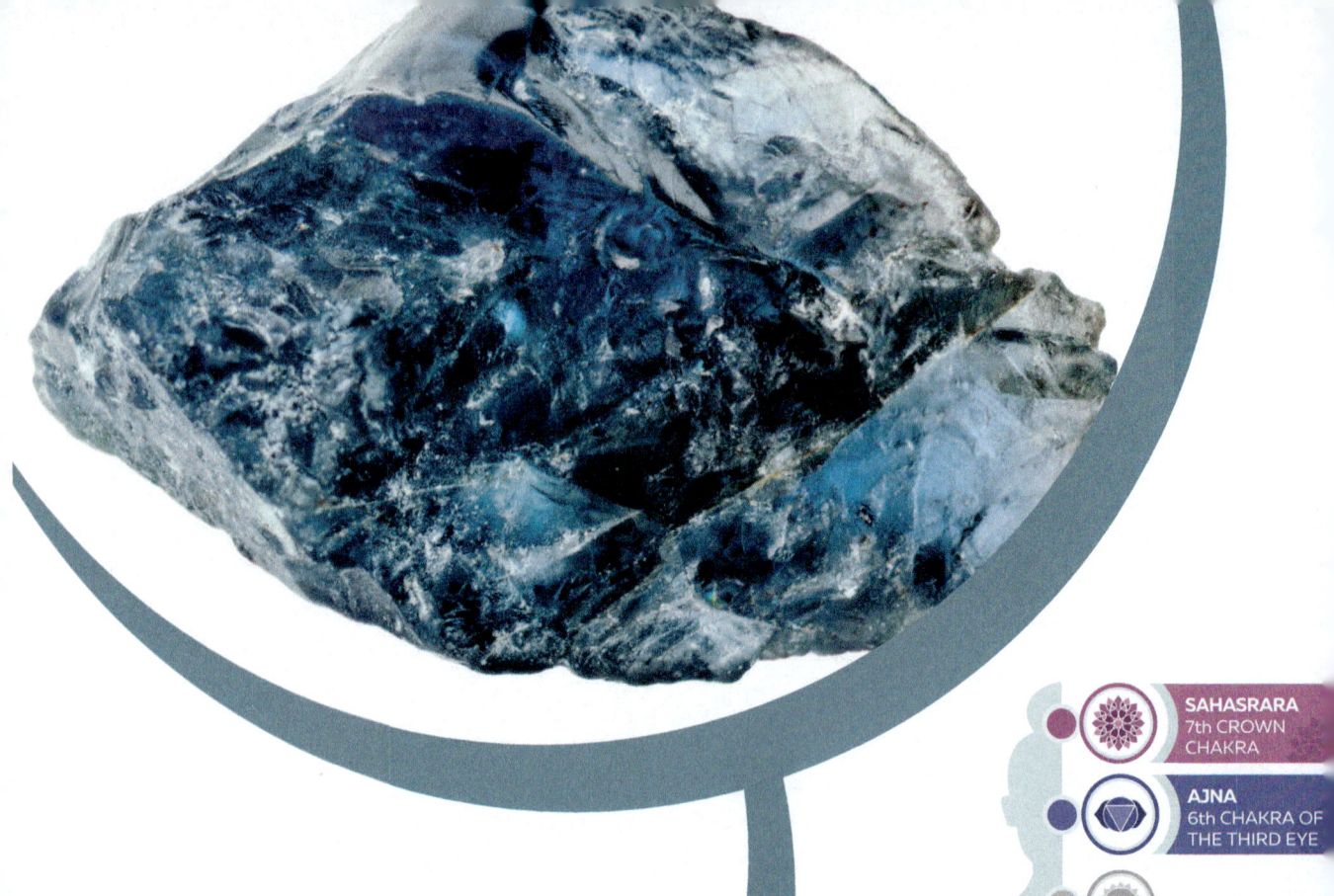

Sapphire

Colors:
Blue

Crystal structure:
Trigonal

Zodiac sign:
Gemini, Libra

SAHASRARA
7th CROWN CHAKRA

AJNA
6th CHAKRA OF THE THIRD EYE

108

History:
It is related to a fairy tale about the 3 sons of the King of Serendib (present-day Sri Lanka) who, intent on wandering the world, fortuitously discover a mine chock-full of sapphires. Hence the English term "Serendipity" was born, meaning "lucky discovery of something beautiful and unexpected."

Properties:
Suitable for those who are seeking personal growth and need to elevate their spirits but also to experience reality in a balanced way, it helps us put our thoughts and emotions in order.

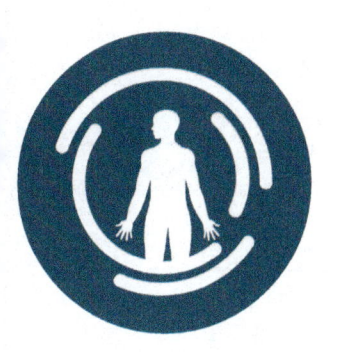

Body benefits:
Helps reduce body temperature in case of fever and prevents colds. Strengthens the kidneys and heart and has a beneficial effect on the circulatory system.

Mind and spirit benefits:
Sapphire helps put thoughts and emotions in order, driving away negative and toxic ones. It allows one to develop greater self-control to ward off vices.

How to treat the stone:
To purify it, we can use water, a clay block, fumes from real incense, or an amethyst druse (just place it on top), while to charge it, we can use a quartz druse or simply moonlight.

Zircon

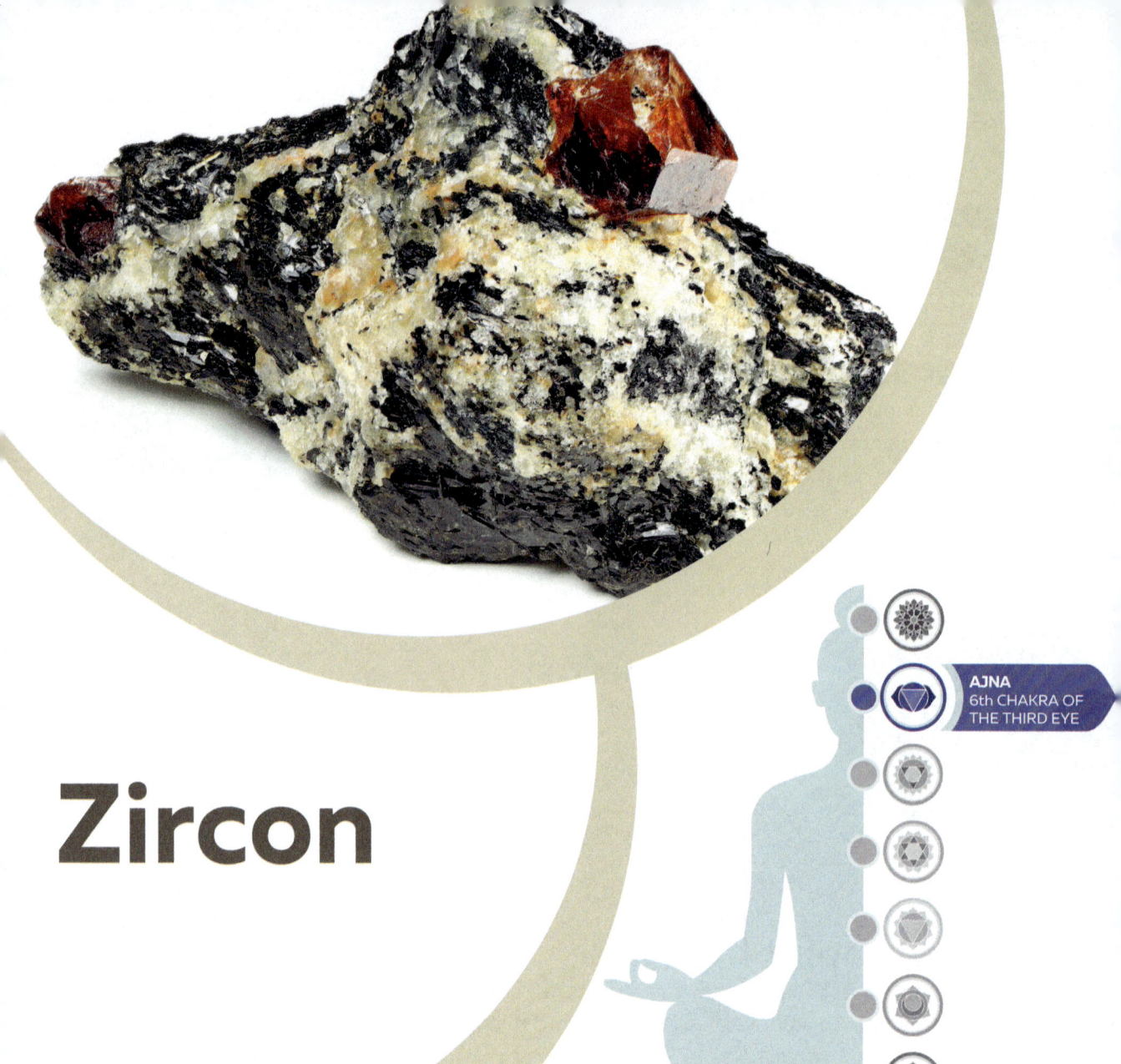

AJNA
6th CHAKRA OF THE THIRD EYE

Colors:
Gray, Orange, Red-Brown, Blue, Colorless

Crystal structure:
Tetragonal

Zodiac sign:
Sagittarius, Scorpio

History:
Legends related to zircon reveal that it was once used to cure madness and ward off evil spirits. Fun fact: The oldest specimen found in Australia dates back 4.4 billion years.

Properties:
It succeeds in freeing us from attachment to material goods and brings our spirituality to a higher level.

Body benefits:
Helps cleanse the liver, spleen, and also endocrine glands. Increases physical strength and gives us vitality and energy.

Mind and spirit benefits:
Helps develop mindfulness, freeing us from obsessive thoughts that plague us.

How to treat the stone:
To purify zircon, we can use salt and water, essential oils such as bach flowers, earth, incense, moonlight, sound, and breath--in short, all the methods we know are fine. To charge it best, instead, we can place it on an amethyst druse or hyaline quartz; moonlight will also work fine.

Conclusion

We have come to the end of this guide, and I hope you have enjoyed it and found it useful.

I would like to remind you that crystal therapy is a holistic treatment that serves to work on the totality of the aspects that form us as human beings: soul, body, and mind, but it cannot replace traditional medicine in any way.

If you liked this guide and I was able to introduce you to the world of crystal therapy, I would ask you to leave a small review on Amazon so we can encourage new projects.

If you don't like something or have any advice for me, I ask you to write me directly in my mailbox:

"keller.ambra@gmail.com"

I will read your suggestions with interest, and they will surely be a cue for me to improve.

I await your positive review on Amazon in the meantime.

Printed in Great Britain
by Amazon